150 YEARS OF NEVADA MEDICINE

(AND MORE)

NEVADA'S MEN AND WOMEN HEALERS

ANTON P. SOHN MD
ROBERT M. DAUGHERTY MD

SECOND EDITION, 2024
RENO, NEVADA

TotalRecall Publications, Inc.
1103 Middlecreek
Friendswood, Texas 77546
281-992-3131 281
www.totalrecallpress.com

Cover: Cover Photograph by the Nevada Historical Society
Front Cover: Dr. James Gerow, Nurses, Indian Mother w/ Newborn
Child held by a Nurse, 1920s

ISBN: 978-1-64883-260-4
UPC: 6-43977-42604-8

1   2   3   4   5   6   7   8   9   10
150 Years of Nevada Medicine
Is Made Possible by a Grant from
The Nevada History of Medicine Foundation, Inc.

Colophon is trademarked

SECOND EDITION (2024)

THIS BOOK IS DEDICATED TO THE

MEN AND WOMEN HEALERS

WHO HAVE PRACTICED MEDICINE IN NEVADA
AND MADE OUR LIVES BETTER

LEND US A HAND
TO RECORD
NEVADA'S HISTORY OF MEDICINE

We have Received Numerous Responses from
Individuals with Information on Doctors and Others
Who have contributed to Nevada's Healthcare
We ask you to Continue this Tradition
To accomplish this Task we ask you to Provide Photographs, Newspaper
Articles, And Personal Information on
Healthcare in Nevada
During the 1800s and the First Half of the 20th Century

Contact:
Anton Sohn MD at antonps@gbis.com

150 Years of Nevada Medicine
Officially approved as a Legacy Project as part of
Nevada's 150th year Celebration

Books by Greasewood Press

Blachley, Anne. *Good Medicine: Four Las Vegas Doctors & the Golden Age of Medicine*. Reno: 2000.

Blachley, Anne. *Pestilence, Politics, and Pizzazz: Public Health in Las Vegas*. Reno: 2002.

Bolstad, Owen. *Larry Nelson, A Doctor Who Cared: The* Story of Laurence D. Nelson, M.D. Reno: 2000. Unpublished.

Cudek, Phyllis and Anton Sohn. *Better Medicine: The History of the University of Nevada School of Medicine*. Reno: 2003.

Montgomery, Payne, Sohn, Thompson and Toole. *Idaho Wildflowers in the River of No Return Wilderness: Medicinal Use, Pistol Creek Ranch History & Geology*. Reno: 2013.

Pugh, Richard. *Cutting Edge: Reflections & Memories of Doctors on Medical Advances in Reno*. Reno: 2002.

Pugh, Richard. *Serving Medicine: The Nevada State Medical Association & The Politics of Medicine*. Reno: 2002.

Pugh, Richard. *Nevada Veterinarians: Profiles of Doctors in a Caring Profession*. Reno: 2007.

Pugh, Richard and Anton Sohn, *The Birthplace of Nevada Medicine: Carson City*. Reno: 2009.

Sohn, Anton, *Hospital Builder: Quincy E. Fortier, A Nevada Physician*. Reno: 1996. Unpublished.

Sohn, Anton *Healers of 19th-Century Nevada*. Reno: 1997.

Sohn, Anton and Carroll Ogren. *People Make The Hospital: History of Washoe Medical Center*. Reno: 1998.

Sohn, Anton Editor. *Frontier Surgeon & Georgetown Medical School Dean: Reminiscences of George Martin Kober, M.D., LL.D. (1850-1931) Vol. II*. Reno: 2007.

Sohn, Anton and Robert Daugherty. *Doctoring in Nevada: Inspiration, Dedication & History*. Reno: 2013.

Sohn, Anton *A Saw, Pocket Instruments and Two Ounces of Whiskey: Frontier Military Medicine in the Great Basin*. Spokane: Arthur Clark, 1998.

Sohn, Anton and Robert Daugherty. *150 Years of Nevada Medicine (and more)*. Reno: 2014 (First Edition).

Books Sponsored by Great Basin Hist. of Medicine

Bolstad, Owen. *Leslie Moren: Fifty Years an Elko Country Doctor.* Reno: University of
    Nevada Oral History Program, 1992.

UNR Oral History program, *Noah Smernoff: A Life in Medicine.* Reno: University of
    Nevada Oral History Program, 1992.

One hundred and twentyone oral histories archived in the Pathology Department at
    UNSOM.

Barker, Eileen, *This Won't Hurt a Bit: Harry Massoth, DDS*. Reno: 1995

CONTENTS

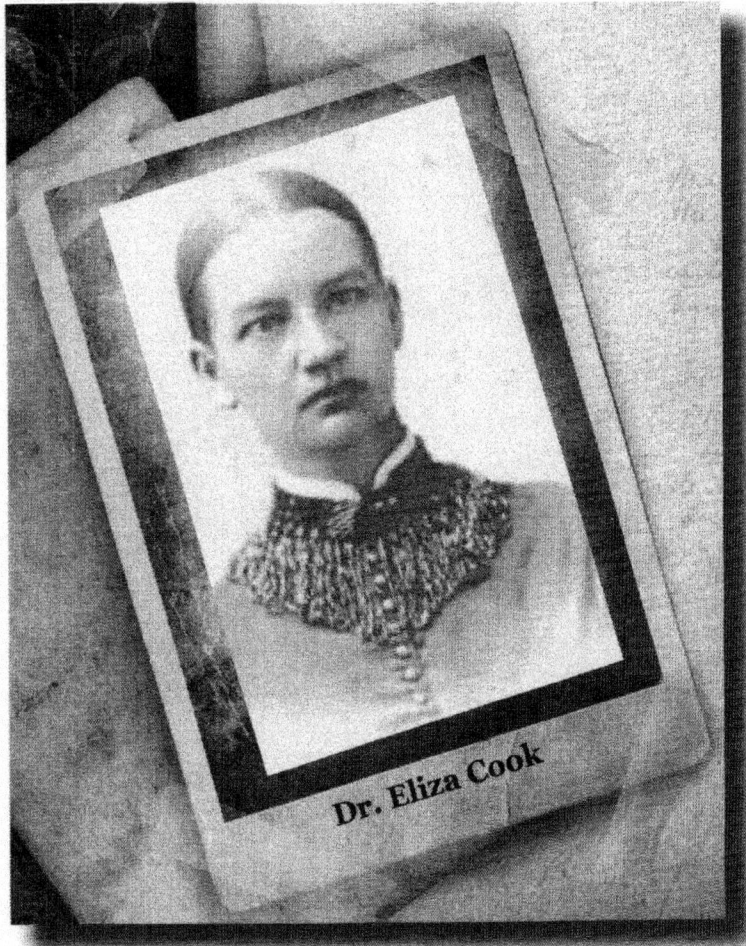

Dr. Eliza Cook

INTRODUCTION
150 YEARS OF NEVADA MEDICINE

Greasewood Tablettes, the Nevada History of medicine Bulletin was established in 1989 to preserve the stories and histories of the men and women who have contributed to Nevada's unique culture by delivering healthcare for over 150 years. A review of *Greasewood Tablettes* shows the richness of Nevada's history of medicine. These articles give insight into we were, and how we got to where we are today. Nevada's recorded medicine history began in in the Utah Territory in 1851 when the first doctor arrived in the community of Mormon Station (Genoa) and continues to the present day with cutting-edge advances of healthcare in Nevada.

The book tells the story of the many parts of Nevada's medical history including the following: Chinese doctors, Native American doctors, midwives, home remedies, medical education, medical doctors, and more. All of these contribute to the fabric of medicine in Nevada. To neglect one diminishes the whole.

These stories and histories of little-known women and men who have developed Nevada's healthcare system and have made important contributions and should not be forgotten or lost in history. The histories highlight the contributions of numerous 'healthcare providers' of all types—hydropaths, homeopaths, shamans, Thompsonians, etc. Their philosophies on treatment and cause of disease, when added to the problem of unregulated medical schools, poor education of doctors, and lack of profession oversight gives us insight into medical care 150 years ago. We use 'healthcare providers' reluctantly because the individuals in this book are not only providers, but also are caring, dedicated, and sacrificing individuals who made our lives better. Retelling their stories will help Nevada's citizens realize their relatives to be remembered. Citizens have stepped forward and called attention to acquaintances who have contributed to Nevada's history. Since the founding of *Greasewood Tablettes*, the editors were pleased to hear from readers with information lost to historians.

This book tell the story of women rising to become equal to men in delivering healthcare to citizens of our state. You will read "Women Doctors in the Nevada" and see that the University of Nevada School of Medicine is playing a part in bringing gender equality to the medical profession. The joint effort of men and women physicians will drive discoveries and new modalities of treating disease.

Telling the story of the history of medicine in Nevada provides an important record. Obviously, all aspects of over one hundred and fifty years of healthcare cannot be recorded in one book, but this book is about the early men and women but who have left an imprint on Nevada. Some left a small fingerprint on the state and were here a short time, while others left a large footprint and made Nevada their home.

ORGANIZATION
150 YEARS OF NEVADA MEDICINE

The volume, number, and year of each issue of *Greasewood Tablettes* is at the end of the article, and the author is listed at the beginning. Initially only articles from *Greasewood Tablettes* were to be included in **150 Years of Nevada Medicine**, but to be complete we were compelled to include additional information. Also, articles not relevant to Nevada were eliminated.

Accordingly this endeavor will be a collection of *Greasewood Tablettes'* articles grouped into eleven chapters: Medical Education, Medical Disciplines/Specialties, Hospitals, Frontier Military Medicine, Native American Medicine, Chinese Medicine, Diseases, The Hood Dynasty, 19th-Century Doctors, 20th-Century Doctors, and The Unusual.

The essays are unchanged from their original publication in *Greasewood Tablettes* except for three considerations. First, we deleted repeat information, although some repetition is necessary to maintain the integrity of the original essay. Second, the titles and some essays were edited to conform to a uniform design, but they still reflect the original content and subject matter. Third, new information is added to increase the scope and completeness of **150 YEARS OF NEVADA MEDICINE**.

AUTHORS

ROBERT M. DAUGHERTY MD

Dr. Robert M. Daugherty has devoted his career to building programs in medical education. He retired in 2004 as Vice President for Health Sciences at the University of South Florida in Tampa. Before South Florida he served twenty-years as the Dean of the University of Nevada School of Medicine (UNRSOM) where he built statewide educational, research, and clinical enterprises. Dr. Daugherty was recruited to Nevada in 1981 after the school transitioned from a two-year to a four-year program. He recruited nationally renowned clinical and basic sciences chairs, developed a clinical campus in southern Nevada, managed hospital relations with public, private, and Veteran Administration Hospital affiliates, built strong rural outreach programs, and oversaw the development of statewide residency programs.

After Dr. Daugherty retired from UNRSOM, the University of South Florida recruited him to become Dean of the College of Medicine and Vice President for Health Sciences, where he oversaw three colleges–Medicine, Nursing, and Public Health–as well as the university's relationships with its major affiliated hospitals.

Well-known for his roles in shaping national issues relevant to medical education, Dr. Daugherty served as chairman of the Council of Deans of the Assoc. of Amer. Med. Colleges (aamc), where he spearheaded its leadership development program to prepare academicians to become deans. He was also on the aamc's Advisory Panel on the Mission and Organization of Medical Schools.

While involved in the Amer. Med. Assoc. (AMA), Dr. Daugherty served three elected terms on the ama Council on Med. Education, which he chaired in 1998-1999. He served as an UNRSOM representative on the Liaison Committee on Med Education(lcme), which he chaired for two years, and served as the ama's representative to the board of the National Board of Medical Examiners (nbme). In 2002, he served on the Institute of Medicine's Committee on Introducing Behavioral and Social Sciences into Medical School Curricula.

With faculty from Nevada and Florida, Dr. Daugherty was active in international efforts to set standards for the quality of medical education and to establish the Council of Rectors for the Central Asian Republics. Their work was funded by the American International Health Alliance through the U.S. Agency for International Development.

Dr. Daugherty is a University of Kansas graduate, with an undergraduate major in chemistry, and an MD from its medical school in 1960. He was Associate Dean for Education at Indiana University SOM from 1978-81 and was responsible for medical student education, graduate medical education (residencies) and Continuing Medical Education (CME). He and his deceased wife, Sandra, were honored as the 2004 University of Kansas Medical School Alumni of the Year.

ANTON P. SOHN MD

Dr. Anton P. Sohn graduated from Indiana University School of Medicine in 1961, interned at San Francisco City and County Hospital, and completed a residency in pathology in Tacoma, Washington, with one of the country's foremost forensic pathologist, Dr. Charles P. Larson. Captain Sohn served in the U.S. Army in Vietnam as Chief of Pathology of the Ninth Medical Laboratory in Saigon where he was awarded the Bronze Star for Meritorious Service Under Hostile Fire.

After discharged from the U.S. Army, Dr. Sohn came to Reno in 1968 to pursue a career in pathology. At Washoe Medical Center (Renown Regional Medical Center) appointed director of the laboratory, founded the hospital's Pulmonary Function Laboratory, and served on its Board of Governors.

Dr. Sohn is a strong supporter of organized medicine. In 1977, he was president of Washoe County Medical Society (wcms) and in 1984 president of the Nevada State Medical Association (nsma). It was during his active participation in nsma that he became interested in Nevada's medical history after hearing stories of the 'old days' by nsma leaders. Sohn received the Nevada Physician of the Year award in 1991, and he received the President's Award for Service to Medicine in 1998 and 2011.

Dean Daugherty recruited Dr. Sohn, a member of Reno pathologists with twenty members, to be chairman of pathology at UNRSOM in 1984. (Doctors Sam Parks, Roger Ritzlin, and Sohn lead the department for twenty-five-years.) In the department Dr. Sohn founded the UNRSOM Cytogenetics Laboratory with Bill McKnight of Sierra Nevada Laboratories. He also founded the Great Basin History of Medicine Program. As part of the program, Doctors Owen Bolstad and Sohn started the UNRSOM oral history archives in the department of pathology. Several chapters in this book are the result of this endeavor. For example: The Great Carlin Canyon Train Wreck and Adventure in the High Sierra.

Doctors Bolstad and Sohn founded *Greasewood Tablettes,* A quarterly history of medicine bulletin and Greasewood Press. The press has published fourteen books on the history of medicine. Dr. Sohn also was the Nevada Editor for the *Western Journal of Medicine* and a research associate at the Johns Hopkins Institute of the History of Medicine.

The use of the name *Greasewood* in the history of medicine program is an interesting story. Dr. S.N. 'Nick' Landis, Reno's first oncologist, frequently stopped by Dr. Sohn's office at wmc to chat and sometimes consult on a patient.

On one occasion Dr. Landis told Dr. Sohn about an Indian man referred to him by a Fallon Clinic doctor. The man had metastatic melanoma to the liver. Dr. Landis told the patient the cancer was incurable, and he had nothing to offer and told him, "Go back to

Fallon, get your life in order, and see your medicine man." One year later the patient came back to thank Dr. Landis for referring him to the medicine man. After an examination and finding no evidence of tumor, Dr. Landis asked him about his treatment. He was told that the medicine man told him to daily drink tea made from the leaves of the Greasewood Bush (also known as the Creosote Bush). Further research revealed that for over twelve thousand years Great Basin Indigenous People have used all parts of greasewood for medicinal purposes. The upshot of this information resulted in a clinical study by the biochemistry department at UNSOM, and no anti-neoplastic (anti-cancer) properties were found in the plant to explain the tumor regression.

After Dr. Sohn suggested the name Greasewood, Dr. Bolstad added the name Tablettes, French for tablets to give the quarterly bulletin sophistication.

LETTER: 1989 EDITOR OF THE
PREMIER ISSUE OF
GREASEWOOD TABLETTEs

Anton P. Sohn MD

Since 1985, we have given sophomore medical students a perspective on the history of medicine by requiring them to write research paper on the history of a disease. Dr. Fred Anderson also had an interest in history of medicine and gave priceless articles of historical significance to the library at the School of Medicine.

There has been no organized continuing effort to record and preserve the medical history of our state. Unless we soon develop a centralized source for publishing and preserving items of historical interest, we will lose these valuable items of our history. As a result I approached Dean Robert Daugherty who endorsed the concept and authorized the formation of a section of medical history in the department of pathology, which we named the Great Basin History of Medicine Program. The program was formed with the help of Martha Hildreth PhD, and Bruce Moran PhD, from unr's History Department, and Tom King PhD, from the oral history section.

We will publish a bulletin, *Greasewood Tablettes*, on a regular basis with historical information relating to medicine in our state. We will accumulate material to be published by the University Press. Also we will develop a central agency for collection of photographs, artifacts, manuscripts, documents, records, and other such memorabilia. This material will provide a valuable source for any future author or researcher and establish a permanent record of our medical history.

There have been previous efforts both by individuals and local and county historical societies to preserve our history. We solicit your opinions and ideas as to how to proceed with this project, and we would appreciate any assistance you might give Dr. Owen Bolstad, a retired member of our department, to help with this project. You can write him at the department of pathology with any questions or suggestions.

This new program of medical history cannot hope to expand and develop without the support of the medical community and interested individuals. We solicit your comments, criticisms, ideas, suggestions, and ask for your support of our program.

Premier Issue, Winter 1989

ILLUSTRATIONS

CHAPTER I:
MEDICAL EDUCATION

After WWII and the establishment of the National Institute of Health (NIH), bio-medical research became prominent in our country's medical schools, which led to an increased emphasis on specialties, and as a result many doctors moved away from primary care.

With the enactment of the 'Great Society' program to make the latest research available to benefit the public, it became clear that there was a shortage of primary care physicians in our communities. This realization led the U.S. Congress to provide funds for the development of new medical schools in 1960s and '70s. As a result, over twenty new community-based medical schools were established with the goal of training physicians in a community setting similar to where they were needed.

The development of community based medical schools in the U.S. was in response to the 'Great Society's War on Poverty by President Lyndon B. Johnson. The 1964 program is described as the largest social improvement agenda since President Franklin D. Roosevelt's 'New Deal.'

In October 1965, the Heart Disease, Cancer, and Stroke Act by the U.S. Congress, authorizing the establishment and maintenance of regional medical programs, became law. Its purpose was to make the latest advances from bio-medical research available to the American people. The act provided for the creation of two programs in Nevada: one in Reno headed by Dr. Dave Roberts, and another in Las Vegas led by Dr. Hugh Follmer. Their objectives were to see that each Nevada hospital had the latest medical journals and continued medical education (CME). Dr. George Smith also helped with the program, which gave him opportunities to lobby throughout the state for a medical school in Nevada.

The Nevada Legislature created the University of Nevada School of Medical Sciences (UNSOMS) in 1969. From 1971 to 1977 the initial classes were taught basic sciences in a two-year program, and they got get clinical training at another medical school. Therefore, after two years at UNSOM they had to transfer to a MD degree-granting program at another school. In 1977, the school became a four-year MD degree-granting institution and became the University of Nevada Reno School of Medicine. The first class graduated as medical doctors in 1980, but they still had to get postgraduate training in another state.

UNRSOM, a designated a community-based medical school, is defined by the Association of Medical Colleges as a medical school that does not have an integrated teaching hospital. The School received full accreditation in 1972 and is a non-federal school.

Thus, UNRSOM was established as part of a national priority to increase the number of primary care physicians. When the Nevada Legislature authorized the medical school to become a four-year MD program, they specified four objectives:

- Create opportunity for Nevada students to study medicine
- Provide primary care physicians for rural Nevada
- Provide cme for practicing physicians
- Promote primary care training

After forty-four years UNRSOM is meeting these objectives, but recent laws passed by the U.S. Congress make it necessary for UNSOM to increase its enrolment in order to meet the increased demand for doctors in Nevada and in the U.S. According to the AMA and John Packham, an administrator at UNRSOM, in 2014 Nevada has 2.24 physicians per 1,000 residents, which compares to 3.27 per 1,000 for the U.S. In other words, Nevada needs 2,829 new physicians to meet the national average.

TEACHER TO REMEMBER
PETER FRANDSEN, PhD

Peter Frandsen's autobiography edited by Anton P. Sohn MD

The editors of the Great Basin History of Medicine have been meeting with senior physicians from Nevada to select subjects for its continuing series of oral history recordings. After interviewing a number of these candidates, we noticed a striking coincidence. In conversations with older doctors, almost without exception, Dr. Peter Frandsen was mentioned.

Peter Frandsen, a native of Denmark, came to Reno with his parents at an early age. He received a BS degree from the University of Nevada in 1895, where he studied human anatomy, physiology, and histology with the intent of studying medicine. After graduating from UN he took a job with a borax mining company, locating borax and soda deposits in the deserts of northwestern Nevada. Later, he took a job teaching in a 'ungraded school' in central Nevada to save money for his education.

Dr. Cowgill, one of his instructors at the UN urged Frandsen to apply to Harvard University and secure a degree there before entering medical school. Dr. Cowgill's letters to Harvard gained Frandsen admission to that University as a sophomore without examination, and at the end of his first year, he advanced to senior standing. This was truly remarkable, since at that time the UN had not received full academic recognition, and Frandsen had no high school credentials.

Graduating from Harvard with an AB degree, he intended "to study medicine, but was persuaded to continue graduate work at Harvard with the offer of a teaching fellowship. He served for some time as a laboratory instructor in comparative anatomy at Harvard and in general zoology at Radcliffe College. He had completed some thirty units toward a PhD at Harvard when, in 1899, Dr. J.E. Stubbs, president of the UN, visited Peter Frandsen in Cambridge, and offered him a position. To fill this position, Frandsen needed to acquire some experience with animal diseases and arrangements were made for him to study at the Bureau of Animal Industry in Washington, DC, during the ensuing summer.

Frandsen returned to Reno in 1900 in the midst of an anthrax epidemic in the Truckee Meadows. Fortunately, with the experience he had gained in Washington, he easily diagnosed the disease with a microscope and cultures in his laboratory. He became assistant professor of zoology and bacteriology. For at least four summers, he and another biology professor spent weeks gathering botanical and zoological specimens. These expeditions, for the most part, were spent on horseback with a pack train in Elko County. It was during these trips that he developed his deep appreciation for Nevada. He was also teaching psychology. In 1909, he was granted sabbatical leave to travel and study in Europe for a year.

During those early years, Professor Frandsen developed a close association with the medical profession. Many of the local physicians felt the need for help in diagnosing infectious diseases and pathology and turned to Frandsen and his laboratory, where microscopes, slide preparations, cultures, and laboratory animals were available. Frandsen worked closely with the local doctors and developed many close friendships.

He mentions many of the early doctors in his reminiscences, but singles out Dr. W.H. Hood as perhaps his closest friend. Frandsen went on frequent vacation trips with Dr. Hood. They loved to go camping, fishing, or simply travelling. On these trips they met many old friends and made new friends. Frandsen tells of one trip when a filling station attendant came limping out with his hand on his back. Dr. Hood asked the man what his trouble was, and he replied that his kidneys were hurting. Hood told him to raise his arms, and began thumping on the man's back. Soon, Hood exclaimed, "Kidneys nothing! What you have is a low-grade pneumonia from the flu. Here, make up this plaster. Put it on your back when you go to bed, and you'll be all right." The man asked, "Are you a doctor? What do I owe you?" Dr. Hood replied, "Not a damned cent, I'm on vacation."

Sometime later, there was a typhoid epidemic in Reno, which was later, traced to a dairy. During the epidemic, which caused great alarm in the community, Professor Frandsen, together with Dr. O.P. Johnstone of the State Hygienics Laboratory, prepared a vaccine against typhoid, and announced it to the public in an effort to allay the concern. To prove the safety of the vaccine, they gave each other extra-large doses and promptly suffered rather "vigorous reactions."

Frandsen, a member of the National Social Hygiene Association, lectured frequently against the anti-vivisectionists, and gave lectures on venereal disease. As one of his duties with the Animal Experiment Station, he staged Farmers' Institutes all over Nevada, and became acquainted with physicians, farmers, and ranchers statewide. He was a director and almost perpetual vice president of the Nevada Tuberculosis And Health Association.

Frandsen continued to be active both in scholastic and medical affairs. He was instrumental in the formation of the Student Health Service at the University and together with LeRoy Fothergill, organized a premedical honorary society named Omega Mu Iota. This society later became affiliated with the national premedical honors society, Alpha Epsilon Delta. He gave several scientific papers before WCMS physicians and was frequently invited to attend their meetings.

After returning from his sabbatical in Europe he lectured to WCMS on the subject of 'Insect-Borne Protozoan Diseases' with slides collected from laboratories in Rome, Paris, Berlin, and London.

He was invited to present several papers at NSMA meetings on the subject of hemophilia, and on another occasion on the subject of the Mendelian Inheritance of Night Blindness. In 1924, the University of Nevada granted him an honorary Doctor of Law.

Peter Frandsen rather drifted into the directorship of the premedical program at the UN, and it is because of this program that Dr. Frandsen became best known. Since 1895 several hundred premedical students from the University of Nevada have graduated, and the majority of them become physicians. A considerable number became dentists, veterinarians, morticians, and many others have went on to earn degrees in biology or botany in preparation for careers in the teaching profession. His students have earned positions in the Biological Survey, the National Park Service, and the U.S. Forestry Service.

Dr. Frandsen, to whom his students fondly referred as 'Professor Bugs,' was widely known throughout the academic world. He took a personal interest in each of his students, carefully evaluating their abilities and guiding them in their studies. When he wrote a letter of recommendation to a medical school, the student could be virtually assured of acceptance.

His students have received MD degrees from at least twenty-one medical schools in the United States. Frandsen was particularly proud of the fact that at least twelve sons of local physicians took their premedical studies with him and went on to become doctors.

Many testimonials to the influence of Peter Frandsen can be found within the memoirs of his students. In his honor the Agriculture Building, constructed in 1918, was named the Peter Frandsen Humanities Building. A bronze plaque in his honor, commissioned by his former students, is inscribed with the names of seventy-one of those students. The plaque is displayed at the entrance to the Doctors Hood History of Medicine Library.

Most of these students are well-known and respected physicians and dentists in the community. Among his many other honors Frandsen was given the Distinguished Nevadan Award in 1958. On several occasions, he was offered positions at other institutions, with the promise of higher pay and greater research opportunities, but his love of Nevada led him to decline the offers. Dr. Frandsen retired in 1942 as Professor of

Biology and Head of the Department of Zoology. He moved to Oroville, California, and operated an olive orchard until his death in 1967.

EDITORS' NOTE:

Anthrax is a bacterium that is found in soil. It can be deadly to animals and humans. In addition, the bacterium has the ability to form spores and exists in a dormant form and be reactivated years later. Reference: An undated typewritten autobiography by Dr. Frandsen and given to Dr. Fred Anderson.

Vol. II, No. 4, Spring 1992

MEDICAL EDUCATION
THE BEGINNING

T. Scully and G.T. Smith:

The University of Nevada has been preparing students for careers in health sciences since college level courses were first offered in 1887, but only in the last forty to fifty years have health and science programs grown to maturity.

After World War II there was a dramatic population increase in the Nevada, and in the 1950s an almost 100 percent increase, which lead to the identification of some serious healthcare deficiencies. A medical technology program had been established in 1950, and a college program in nursing education had been approved by the legislature. After the university received a gift of $100,000 from A.E. Orvis, the Orvis School of Nursing was established, and the first class of nursing students started in 1957. A study done by the Western Interstate Commission on Higher Education (WICHE) suggested that Nevada should begin planning for a two-year medical school. The proposal to establish a medical school stirred great controversy within the State.

Should the school be a two-year school, with students finishing their medical educations in out-of-state, degree granting medical schools, or should it be a full four-year school in Nevada.

The proposed location of the school in Reno further evoked the long-standing rivalry between northern and southern factions of the state. The largest issue was financial, however, for with a population of fewer than 400,000, many taxpayers felt the state could just not afford a medical school. In February 1967, Reno philanthropist H. Edward Manville, Jr., announced a gift of $1 million to the University of Nevada Medical School. This offer was later followed by a promise from industrialist Howard Hughes to provide up to $6 million for the medical school.

These gifts broke the deadlock, and on January 11, 1969, the University Board of Regents approved a two-year medical school for the Reno campus. On March 25, 1969, Governor Paul Laxalt signed into law AB 130, which appropriated $58,000 for startup expenses. On March 26, the *Nevada State Journal* carried the following story: "Governor

Paul Laxalt signed AB 130 allowing the UN Board of Regents to establish a health sciences program, including a medical school, at the University of Nevada, Reno." The issue split the legislature and the Board along sectional lines since a feasibility study was proposed in 1967. That battle ended temporarily when Howard Hughes pledged up to $6 million over twenty years to the school.

Strong opposition remained as the plan was broadened from the original two-year medical school concept to include related studies and fields. It squeezed through both houses with supporters saying the plan would fill a big need in the State and opponents saying the State could not afford it. The bill would appropriate about $58,000 from the State general funds to get the program off the ground. It also would authorize the Regents to spend about $418,000 in university fees and grants to remodel two old buildings, which have been scheduled for demolition.

Pathologist George T. Smith, who had been director of the Laboratory of Pathophysiology at the Desert Research Institute, became the founding dean.

Dr. Smith was involved in WICHE studies and planning for the new school.

The initial proposal for a two-year medical school had been broadened by the UN Board of Regents to provide two-year basic science education to a variety of pre-professional students. These included pre-dentistry, medical technology, health education, physical therapy, speech pathology, pre-pharmacy and audiology, therefore the institution was named the UN School of Medical Sciences.

Within a few months the school had received grants totaling more than $900,000 from the Commonwealth Fund and the W.K. Kellogg Foundation. In the next year foundation grants totaled $1.2 million, and more than $1.4 million was secured from a variety of federal agencies, in addition to nearly $400,000 raised from local sources.

The charter class of thirty-two students at UNSOMS began their studies in the fall of 1971. The initial faculty numbered nine full-time and five part-time instructors. Many local physicians, who volunteered their time, supplemented this slim cadre. During the first few years, more than two hundred practicing physicians from throughout the state participated in the teaching program, and twenty additional basic science faculty members were recruited.

During the first five years of operation, UNSOMS admitted 221, nineteen from out-of-state and the remainder from Nevada. During those first five years, there were only six dropouts or failures. All of the remaining 215 transferred to degree granting medical schools, and all 215 were granted MD degrees.

EDITORS' NOTE:

Reference: "School of Medical Sciences, University of Nevada." Dr. Tom Scully succeeded Dr. Smith as Dean in 1977, but resigned in 1979 for health reasons.

Vol. I, No. 2, Spring 1990.

COMMUNITY OUTREACH
AND EDUCATIONAL PROGRAMS

Caroline Ford, UNSOM Assistant Dean and Director, 1983-2011

The mid-1960s in Nevada launched the Division of Interdisciplinary Health Sciences that eventually spawned the Nevada State Office of Rural Health within the School of Medicine. The Interdisciplinary Health Sciences Division predated the establishment of the University of Nevada School of Medicine two-year training program in 1967. This division set the tenure of community based medical education and reached out into rural Nevada to recruit candidates that eventually returned to their hometowns to practice medicine.

The School of Medicine introduced a wide array of programs that examined the health workforce needs of the state, technical assistance to clinics and hospitals in medically underserved communities, and economic development issues affecting health care. Additional focus on obstetrical services to isolated communities and partnering with the federal government to diffuse National Health Service Corps candidates continued to respond to pressing health care needs. The Nevada State Office of Rural Health, that became the School of Medicine's link to the state's rural counties, fulfilled many roles to advocate for rural and frontier communities and successfully maintained their distinction as one of the longest operating Offices in the country.

Dr. DeWitt "Bud" Baldwin, founding Program Director, 1971-1983: I think of my years at the UNRSOM and in Nevada as the best years of my life—the most creative, challenging, stimulating and enjoyable. I created the Office of Rural Health in large part because it was obvious that if we were to get the state's support for a four-year medical school, we had to make rural health a priority. I also saw the need to assist small towns to secure adequate health services.

Twenty years after President Johnson's Great Society in the 1960s, the mid-1980s brought a time of tremendous growth nationally for healthcare programs, and in Nevada, UNRSOM led the way with the creation of a statewide Area Health Education Center (AHEC) program. The program's objective, met through community and academic educational partnerships, was to address the interdisciplinary education of healthcare providers, including medical students, and give them experience in medically underserved areas throughout Nevada. The state provided funding with an appropriation in 1987, and was awarded federal funding later that same year. UNRSOM established AHEC centers in Reno, LV and Elko.

The Elko AHEC Center was considered the most frontier and remote in the nation, and it led the way with successful training programs that demonstrated the heart of the program, which made a bridge between an academic medical center and the community.

Recognizing regional healthcare needs by working with community-based boards of directors, UNRSOM created clinical exposures for its students and diffused physicians and other health professionals to areas of need. Medical residency expansions were also a result of the AHEC program; two of the most recent are a "one plus two" rural family medicine residency in Winnemucca in which the 1st year is served in Las Vegas, the final two in Winnemucca, and another resident training program in internal medicine in Elko.

Through AHEC, UNRSOM provided leadership and expanded access to get health career education to hiv/aids and geriatric patients. The Nevada Area aids Education and Training Center was created in 1989 with federal funds to the Center for Education and Health Services Outreach. The science of hiv/aids care progressed so rapidly that it was imperative for a network of expert scientists, clinicians and educators be assembled to educate the health care community about hiv care. By 1992, there were over 1,000 cases of aids in Nevada; however, by 2010 pharmaceutical aids into a chronic condition research and treatment of the disease turned. The continued need to educate health care professionals on current treatment practices has kept the program relevant to changing management of patient care.

Another step in advancing healthcare education was the Nevada Geriatric Education Center established in October 1992. The Center committed to improving healthcare to older adults through education, information, and resources by UNRSOM faculty and other health professionals.

The Outreach Center went on to develop many more programs and services to the state through the som's commitment. They included: the Office of Medical Education & Professional Development, Emergency Medical Services, Telecommunications/ Telehealth that linked over 50 locations across the state, the Obstetrical Access Program, the Nevada Critical Access Hospital Program, the Nevada Health Service Corps—a loan repayment program for healthcare professionals, the Office of Health Professions Research and Policy, Economic Development and Analyses, Technical Assistance, Policy Analysis, and Publications and Reports that now include a biennial edition of the Nevada Rural and Frontier Data Book and annual Graduate Medical Education Resident reports.

Dr. Robert Daugherty, Dean UNRSOM, 1981-1999: At UNRSOM, we reached out to rural Nevada for important reasons. First, we wanted our future physicians (our students) to understand the problems as well as the positives associated with practicing in a resource scarce rural community. Second, we wanted students who lived in rural communities to understand that medicine was a viable career for them. Third, we wanted physicians in rural Nevada to understand that they were not isolated from mainstream medicine. Using technology, we connected them to information centers and to their professional colleagues. Using good, old-fashioned face-to-face meetings, we learned about their concerns and helped bridge gaps that impeded their ability to serve their patients.

Fourth, we wanted the leaders in rural communities to know that the School of Medicine was a resource for them as well. Access to healthcare is a community issue: recruiting and retaining physicians, building clinics, weathering the rise in physician malpractice rates, keeping the hospital viable–all of these community issues were concerns we set out to address through the School of Medicine's Office of Rural Health.

Caroline Ford, Assistant Dean and Director, 1983-2011, Center for Education and Health Services Outreach: History teaches that most events are cyclical, and that people, services, and programs come and go, and then return again. What I learned early on about the "boom and bust" cycle of rural economies was that healthcare would be one of the constants in the community. Some of the practitioners would live, practice their careers and eventually pass on in their communities.

Facilities would be built, age and then be replaced. Services would wax and wane with the demographics and the introduction of new technologies. What seems to have never changed is the spirit of the rural community, the bond of the generational family, the richness of friendships, the common connections of ranchers, miners, cowboys and casino workers. We aspire to improve healthcare services and the quality of life in Nevada as our mission in public health within the School of Medicine. We also live and raise our children in the communities we serve. Our patients and colleagues are our neighbors and friends. This is what makes the difference in our bond with healthcare and our resolve to continue evolving in addressing ever changing needs.

FATHER OF THE MEDICAL SCHOOL
DR. FRED ANDERSON

Dr. Fred M. Anderson was born in 1906 and raised in eastern Nevada on a ranch in the Ruby Mountains. He related that he was a cowboy before working in a pharmacy in the small town of Ruth. According to his oral history, recorded by the University of Nevada Oral History Program, he passed the state pharmacy board examination, "worked one day as a pharmacist" and then attended the University of Nevada in Reno. There, he came under the influence of Professor Peter Frandsen who persuaded him to study medicine.

After graduation in 1928 Anderson was awarded a Rhodes scholarship to Oxford University. Fred returned to the United States and medical school at Harvard where he graduated *cum laude*. A military veteran, he returned after WWII to his roots in Nevada.

There might have been others who earlier thought Nevada should have a medical school, but Fred had the vision and the position to make it happen. In the early 1960s he was chairman of the University of Nevada Board of Regents and a member of WICHE. The commission was composed of three representatives from each of the western states without a medical school. It initiated a feasibility study for a medical school in one of these states, and Nevada, under Dr. Anderson's leadership, was selected.

The finished feasibility study was presented to the UN Board of Regents in a contentious meeting on February 11, 1967. Chairman Fred Anderson relinquished the gavel, stepped down, and fired the 'shot heard around the state.' His motion fueled the *north-south* fight that continues to this day to haunt Nevada. It pitted a surging growth of Las Vegas and Clark County against the established tradition of the north. Anderson moved to form a two-year school of basic medical sciences, taking the first class in the fall of 1971 or 1972. It passed six to two.

For his role in the drama of creating the University of Nevada School of Medicine, Anderson was named the 'Father of the Medical School.' Furthermore, the first building in the School's complex is the Fred M. Anderson Building. In addition to his role in education, Fred had a sense of history that was uncommon. As he traveled around the state consulting on medical cases, he amassed a collection of 19th-century medical instruments, antique books, Indian artifacts, and items related to ranching.

Fred never forgot his ranching background and time in the saddle. His extensive collection of Nevada branding irons was an exhibit at the Nugget in Sparks. It has been said that (when Dr. Anderson asked for a branding iron to be donated for historical preservation, it was not refused. The History of Medicine Library in the new Pennington Education Building on the Reno campus exhibits some of Anderson's collection.

It would be incomplete to relate the above information without saying something about Dr. Anderson as a physician. Attorney Ralph Denton who practiced in Las Vegas and served on the advisory committee to the dean of the medical school was a good friend of Dr. Anderson. Mr. Denton recalled when his son had a fatal burn and Dr. Anderson heard of the accident, he immediately traveled to Las Vegas to comfort the family and treat the boy. He wouldn't take a penny in payment. Governor Mike O'Callaghan summed it by saying, "Anderson was extremely intelligent, but also compassionate."

Vol. XIV, No. 1, Spring 2003

NEVADA'S SCHOOL OF MEDICINE
COMES OF AGE FORTY YEARS

Anne McMillin, UNSOM Public Relations Director

The final week of September 2009 witnessed a flurry of celebratory activity aimed at recognizing the fortieth anniversary of the University of Nevada School of Medicine with a series of events to pay tribute to the successes of the medical school since its establishment in 1969.

School of Medicine Founding Dean George Smith invited all thirty-two members of the charter class, which entered in the fall of 1971, to gather at the home of Mrs. Nena Miller, widow of N. Edd Miller, unr President when the School started, to get reacquainted and discuss their medical careers and life paths since completing their first two years of medical school basic sciences in 1973. About a dozen members of that class, their spouses, and inaugural and current faculty members attended the September 23 reception.

The next night the twenty-eightieth annual University of Nevada, Reno Foundation Banquet turned its focus to health sciences with a record crowd of nearly 1,000 people coming out to honor the University of Nevada School of Medicine's 40th anniversary at John Ascuaga's Nugget in Sparks.

University President Milton Glick delivered a big announcement when he revealed that the William N. Pennington Foundation committed $10 million for the purpose of the planned Health Sciences Building, which will allow for the eventual doubling of both the nursing and medical student class sizes when it is complete in the fall of 2011. The building will be named the William N. Pennington Health Science Building and will sit just east of the current Pennington Medical Education Building.

Glick also mentioned the gifts provided for the building from the Nell J. Redfield Foundation and the Thelma B. and Thomas P. Hart Foundation and the many people and organizations that helped the University reach its $15 million goal.

President Glick recognized Dr. George Smith, the founding dean of the medical school, and Dr. Susan Desmond-Hellmann, 1982 UNRSOM graduate. Dr. Desmond-Hellmann is chancellor of the University of California San Francisco and recipient of the School of Medicine's first Outstanding Alumni Award from the School's Alumni Association, which was presented earlier in the evening at a reception. (Dr. Desmond-Hellmann was appointed ceo of the Bill and Melinda Gates Foundation in 2014.)

Distinguished surgeon, teacher, and writer Atul Gawande, staff member of Boston's Brigham and Women's Hospital, gave the keynote address, noting that the challenge for the medical profession today is to make the medical experience better for patients who have long struggled with medicine.

Legislators Joe Dini, Don Mello, and Virgil Getto, who helped establish the school, were recognized with plaques at the reception before the banquet. Dr. George Furman, the first ob/gyn chair in Reno, as well as Dr. Ron Pardini, who taught biochemistry to the first class, attended the festivities. Ted Bacon and Janice Goodhue, two of the original members of the School's advisory board, were at the banquet. Charter faculty member Phil Gillette as well as Georgia Fulstone and Andrea Pelter, early strong supporters of the school attended. Former Deans Robert Daugherty and Steve McFarlane attended the events.

Charter Class members P. Colletti, L. Noble, J. Calvanese, Henry Prupas, J. Moren, E. Piercznski, R. Ainsworth, R. Priest, J. Chamberlain, George Manning, Henry Nelson, and Mark Rhodes attended some or all of the week's events.

The week's festivities concluded September 25 in the Manville auditorium at which current School of Medicine faculty members gave presentations for cme credit to the attendees.

Vol. XX, No. 3, Fall 2009

UNRSOM TWENTIETH ANNIVERSARY

Lynne D. Williams, UNSOM Assist. Public Relations Director

On March 25, 1969, Nevada Assembly Bill 130 establishing the two-year school was signed into law. The charter class entered the program in 1971, and four succeeding classes, completed their basic science studies in Reno. These students then transferred to four-year programs at other medical schools for their clinical years.

According to Dr. Frederick M. Anderson, during those years the government changed its attitude about support of two-year programs, and offered $2.5 million to the medical school to help in its conversion to a four-year, degree-granting institution. The legislature approved the change April 14, 1977, and the school's first class of students to become physicians trained entirely in Nevada graduated in 1980.

The school is now a thriving institution with an annual operating budget of $21 million, approximately half of which is appropriated from the legislature and half is generated through research grants and contracts. Making good on its pledge to serve the needs of the entire state, the school is continually expanding its educational and outreach programs. Although the basic sciences facility and a Family Medicine Center are located on the University of Nevada, Reno campus, four departments are based in Las Vegas and a second Family Medicine Center is housed in a community college building in Las Vegas. Additionally, a new Genetics Network has been established with offices in both Reno and Las Vegas, and this year, the school is planning to buy or construct a building to house the Las Vegas based programs and medical school faculty members.

The latest development in this statewide expansion is Nevada's first kidney transplant program. UNRSOM and University. Medical Center developed this program. Rural communities are important in the school's programs. The Office of Rural Health works with several communities to assess their health needs and to help recruit medical health care professionals. The Area Health Education Center also boosts the health care of rural communities. AHEC is a federally funded program that allows the medical schools to offer continuing education programs for physicians, nurses, and allied health professionals, and to encourage rural students to pursue med. careers.

There are approximately 150 full-time faculty members and more than 600 community physicians who serve as clinical faculty throughout the state. Faculty researchers competed successfully for federal research dollars totaling approximately $3 million each year to investigate some of today's most pressing scientific mysteries: aids and the infections that kill aids patients; stress; hypertension; cancer; Alzheimer's disease; diabetes; and GI disorders.

New equipment and facilities, such as a transmission electron microscope (one of twenty in the nation), a fna synthesizer, a monoclonal antibody laboratory, and a fluorescence imaging system that is one of thirteen in the world allow Nevada's scientists, who have been recruited from prestigious institutions around the country, to continue their research work.

Finally, our students, the proudest measure of the school's success, met–and-exceed national academic standards. As graduates and fully trained physicians, they are filling Nevada's need for doctors, especially in the rural communities.

What is the most satisfying to planners is the conspicuous absence of the question that plagued them in the early years: "Well, do you think the school is going to make it?" The answer is a resounding, "Yes, the dream is a reality."

Since 1980, the University of Nevada School of Medicine has granted MD degrees to 724 graduates. Of these, 212 have returned to practice medicine in Nevada. These statistics show that the School of Medicine is fulfilling its mission of training physicians for our state.

EDITORS' NOTE:

This article originally appeared in the School of Medicine bulletin, *Synapse*, under the titled "School of Medicine Enters Adulthood."

Vol. II, No. 1, Spring 1991

SCHOOL OF MEDICINE'S
1981 BUDGET CRISIS

Robert M. Daugherty MD

In January 1981, I flew into Reno on a sunny cold Sunday from Indiana to meet with the Acting Dean Mazzaferri and his staff, including financial officers, to review the School of Medicine's 1981-'83 budget request to the legislature. The state budget office had already reduced the budget, and we knew a fight was coming. Like the 2008-'09 financial situation, 1981 was a time of economic recession. The following Monday at 6:00 am, President Joe Crowley and I drove to Carson City for my presentation of the medical school's budget to the Nevada Assembly Ways and Means Committee. Chairman Roger Bremmer called the meeting to order and President Crowley introduced me as the new dean. He said more nice things about me in that introduction than he would ever say again.

I started my budget presentation, and no more than two minutes later I was interrupted by someone, who said, "When did we decide to have a medical school?" Committee member Robert Robinson followed this, "This medical school is an albatross around the neck of the state. We would save money by buying every medical student a Ferrari and sending them out of state." Member Jack Verglies quickly followed him, "Dr. Daugherty, I sure hope you haven't sold your house in Indiana." The chairman followed this statement, "I sure hope you haven't bought a house in Nevada."

Without hesitation, Mr. Bob Cashell, Chairman of the Board of Regents at the University stood and said, "If I was in the legislature, I wouldn't have voted for the medical school either."

I heard the quiet voice of President Crowley behind me, "Bob, sit down. Bob, sit down." I sat down and Chairman Bremmer adjourned the committee. Everyone in the room left except me. I sat there somewhat amused by what had happened. I have told this story to a number of folks over the years. They often look horrified and comment, "How awful, how devastating." However, this experience reminded me of my Wyoming experience some 5 years earlier. I was hired by the University of Wyoming in 1976 to start a new medical school in Laramie. In my experiences with the Wyoming Legislature, I found that many of the legislators were surprised to learn that the University of Wyoming had approval for the funding of the new school. That experience taught me that there is always another day in dealing with the legislative process.

Thus, as I sat in the Nevada Senate committee room that cold January 1981 day, I reflected on my political education in Wyoming. I realized that the next step was going to be up to me and me alone. After all, the president and the chairman of the Board of Regents not only had not defended the medical school, but they had left the room. What should I do? In the preceding 6 months, as I visited Reno and the state, I met many physicians, legislators, and community leaders. I had accepted the deanship because I felt there was sufficient support of the school despite much vocal opposition.

On one of these visits, I met Mr. Bob Barengo, Speaker of the Assembly from Reno. Dr. Bob Clift, a Reno physician on the search committee, introduced me to him. In fact, Dr. Clift was the only community physician on the committee. He described himself as the 'token doc' on the search committee. Bob and I developed mutual respect, which was assisted by the fact that we had both graduated from the Kansas University School of Medicine.

I had just met my apparent demise! Therefore, I decided to pay Speaker Barengo a visit. In those days in the Nevada Legislature it was easy and comfortable to walk into a legislators' office and visit or seek help. As I walked into the speaker's office he met me with a smile and a hearty, "Hi Dean, how are you and welcome."

I responded that I was fine, but I had a question. "It is my understanding that you, as speaker, appoint the committee chairs in the assembly. Is that correct?" Mr. Barengo responded, "Yes." I immediately responded, "I think you owe me one." I then described what had transpired in the ways and means committee hearing. The Speaker looked at me and asked with a slight smile, "Do you need any funds for Las Vegas?" I responded, "Yes, what should it be?" Barengo, "You decide but get it to me by tomorrow." Needless to say, I presented a Las Vegas budget of $400,000 to him. When I returned, he said, "Dean, your budget will be approved, all of it, including the Las Vegas funds."

I learned my first and most important political Nevada lesson. Always include both Reno and Las Vegas in my requests to the legislature. I also learned that rural Nevada was another priority. On the other hand, by the time I left my deanship, nineteen years later, rural Nevada was my priority, but it no longer was the legislature's priority. In the remaining days and weeks of the 1981 legislative session, I spent much face-to-face time with members of the Assembly Ways and Means Committee. As a result, by the next legislative session, Mr. Bremmer had become supportive of the school. However, it was not always evident because he had his own way of helping. Another member also had a unique way of helping. Mr. Vergiels, never voted for us, but he never voted against us. Other members were never supportive. For example, Robinson was consistently against all of our proposals.

Little did I realize that this initial Nevada political education would carry me through nine more sessions. The School of Medicine and I enjoyed good support from the succeeding legislative leaders over the following nineteen years, giving us the opportunity to provide Nevada's best and brightest students an excellent medical education–second to none in the country.

Vol. XX, No. 1, Spring 2009

CHAPTER II:
MEDICAL DISCIPLINES
AND SPECIALTIES

The concept of a board for the purpose of establishing qualifications to be a specialist was first proposed in 1908 by Dr. Derrick Vail in his presidential address to the American Academy of Ophthalmology and Otolaryngology. He stated, "I hope that the day will come when we as oculists demand a certain amount of preliminary education and training be enforced before a man may be licensed to practice ophthalmology." However, at the time, the biggest problem was an inadequate number of institutions organized to train specialists in the U.S.

Under the leadership of the Council of Medical Education of the American Medical Association studies were undertaken and reports generated by other invested societies to study and bring to order the issues of graduate medical education. In 1914, the ama produced the first list of approved internships.

In 1920, the ama Council on Medical Education appointed a committee on graduate medical degrees to report on the state of graduate medical education opportunities in the U.S. Also in 1920, the Council on Medical Education organized fifteen different clinical and basic science committees and recommended the preparation necessary to secure expertise in each of the specialties.

The Council published the Essentials of Approved Residencies and Fellowships for the specialties in existence in 1928. The boards of the specialties in this section were dermatology, pathology, and pediatrics, and they were recognized in the 1930s.

In 1932, the ama Section of Dermatology and Syphilology and the American Dermatological Association established the American Board of Dermatology and Syphilology.

Thus, the American Academy of Dermatology became the third sponsor in 1939.

The American Board of Pediatrics was formed by the American Academy of Pediatrics in 1933. Its leadership was not sympathetic with creation of specialty boards. They believed that the certification board was a form of self-aggrandizement. They later changed their opinion and created the American Board of Pediatrics.

In 1936, under the sponsorship of the American Society of Clinical Pathologists and the ama section on pathology and physiology, the American Board of Pathology was established. However, it was 1943 before the ama recognized pathology as the practice of medicine.

Thus, in the 1930s, we moved from a time when a physician could indicate himself as any specialist he preferred without training or expertise to become a specialist by an appropriate board.

In addition to qualifications to be recognized as a medical specialist, we will mention some medical disciplines that contributed to Nevada's medical history. At the start of our conquest to tell the story of Nevada medicine from the beginning, we recognized that the practice of medicine in the 19th-century and into the 20th-century healthcare was more than doctors taking care of patients. Midwives not only delivered babies, but they also took care of the sick and injured when no one else was available. In the 19th-century, the distinction between midwives and doctors was sometimes blurred. You will note in this book that some doctors were also called midwives and midwives called doctors.

Furthermore, the practice of medicine needed structure and organization to control the practice of untrained and unknowledgeable practitioners. In the 1800s, the public was unprotected from unscrupulous practitioners. As a result, the Nevada State Medical Association and county societies came into existence. Other programs developed to provide public health alerts and regulations. Slowly but surely strict discipline developed in the medical profession.

DERMATOLOGY IN RENO

Roderick D. Sage MD

Dermatology is a medical discipline that can be traced to antiquity and is thought by historians to be the oldest medical specialty. The skin, being an external organ and visible to anyone interested, readily presents its afflictions for study and treatment. The fact that so many of those rashes look alike has led to great confusion, which in the course of time has been enhanced by the nomenclature of skin disease. One practice has been to label a disease after some early observer, who gained immortality by attaching his name to a new mystery eruption. Further confusion results when a skin problem may be described with *Greek* or *Latin* whoppers. Here is a relative well-known example–*pityriasis lichenoides et varioliformis acuta*, also known by its eponym as Mucha-Haberman Disease. Perhaps because skin diseases are rarely fatal, dermatology has been considered more of a minor specialty, but to those suffering with a skin problem it is a major issue. And more so if the problem is one of the viral poxes or blistering disease such as pemphigus–serious indeed!

The American Board of Medical Specialties was conceived in the early 1920s and incorporated in 1932. Its initial organization was the American Board of Dermatology and Syphilology. Syphilis was a major cause of skin afflictions before the age of penicillin. The syphilis designation was dropped in the 1960s when penicillin had all but eliminated syphilis. It turned out only a temporary victory because syphilis has made resurgence in the last few years.

Dr. Charles McNitt was the first certified dermatologist to practice in northern

Nevada. He was a medical graduate of Columbia University where he trained in dermatology. He came to Reno in 1946 and practiced until 1957. Dr. Mortimer Falk came to town in 1952 and continued practicing until 2002. He graduated from the Univ. of Michigan School of Medicine and trained in dermatology at the Univ. of Pennsylvania.

The third early skin specialist was your author, Dr. R.D. Sage, who came to Reno from Stanford University in 1958.

In earlier times, the first dermatologists served the northern half of Nevada and a wide swath into northeastern California from Alturas to Bishop. With the retirement of Dr. McNitt in 1957, Dr. Falk had the sole responsibility for the dermatology problems of this large area until Dr. Sage arrived. The situation was stable until the mid-1970s, at which time the population of Nevada and the numbers of new physicians, both specialists and generalists, began to surge. (The population of Reno, Sparks, Carson City, and contingent areas in the mid-1950s was close to 60,000, now it has burgeoned to 300,000, while the state is about 3,000,000.)

Until the last quarter of the 20th-century the numbers of certified American skin specialists was stable at 1,500, and they tended to cluster around larger cities, especially if a medical school was nearby. Recent estimate of American dermatologists approaches 18,000.

Treatment modalities, until the recent twenty years, were rather stable. The most used and dependable was ultraviolet light for inflammatory ailments including acne, psoriasis pityriasis rosea, and many forms of eczema. We also treated acne and stubborn inflammatory dermatoses with X-ray therapy, but this method is now outmoded because of the fear of radiation side effects.

Topical management of skin problems was, and still is, the mainstay of the dermatologist for fifty years. A fair amount of hocus pocus helped in the concoction of our various of potions, lotions, and brews containing mixtures of tar, sulfur, salicylic acid, menthol and phenol, to anchor our therapeutic arsenal in the control of itching and inflammations. In recent years these nasty looking stinky messes have given way to the more tolerable and effective steroid preparations for use both outside and inside the skin.

Currently tranquillizers, antihistamines, and some of the recently developed immune modulating drugs are the mainstay of treatment. There was once a great reliance on dietary measures, the most memorable being the dictum against eating chocolate to control acne. We now know that is mostly nonsense.

The 1970s started with the establishment of UNSOM, a two-year program with thirty-two students and expanded to a four-year MD granting program in 1978. The first class of thirty-six with a MD degree graduated in 1980. With the growth of UNSOM, the facilities in Reno and Las Vegas have developed superb teaching programs.

Reno surgeon Fred Anderson is named the founding father of UNSOM, having been in the forefront of a lengthy struggle for funding from the Nevada Legislature. Ultimately, a multi-year donation from the Howard Hughes Foundation convinced the Legislature to fund the school. Not to be forgotten are the numerous Nevadan physicians and generous lay persons, who helped make the new school possible. The class size has been steady at close to 60 in the last few years. At first males predominated, but in recent years the distribution by sexes is equal.

Initially, most of the medical classes were held on the unr campus and at the Veterans Hospital. The early focus was on the preclinical sciences (anatomy, physiology, pharmacology, pathology, and biochemistry). Introductory clinical courses were offered in surgery, medicine, obstetrics and gynecology, and psychiatry, and believe it or not in dermatology. Dr. Falk and I conducted a rather compact ten-day clinical review in conjunction with the student course in skin physiology. Years later after UNRSOMS students had matriculated elsewhere, we learned that in many cases our offerings were their only dermatological exposure in all of their training.

With the advent of our medical program and its expansion to four years, parallel changes were evident with the growth of Reno.

For the two dermatologists who held the fort for so long (1958-'71) changes were underway. A half of a dozen new skin specialists came to town in the 1970s–Doctors Tom Standlee, Alan McCarty, Steven Billstein, Larry Gardner, Victor Rueckl, and Charles Clemmensen. In the 1980s we welcomed Doctors James Torok and Burdick. The 1990s saw more new faces, but in the current century the floodgates opened. By 2010, twenty-eight dermatologists are available to serve the 300,000 area residents and an equal number of persons in contiguous and mainly rural Nevada and California counties. In keeping with the formation of group practice, Doctors Kevin Kiene and Bret Blackhart in Reno now have an office with seven partners and a modern new building. Dr. Clemmensen in Carson City has followed suit with a four-member group and a substantial building. In addition, several smaller coalitions have formed.

Vol. XXI, No. 3, Fall 2010

Vol. XXII, No. 1, Spring 2011

NEVADA STATE MEDICAL ASSOCIATION
THE BEGINNING

Shirley Kershner, *Reno Evening Gazette*, 1951

The room was a small plain one with a rag rug covering the bare floor. The furniture consisted of a shiny black wood stove in one corner, 2 or 3 straight-backed kitchen chairs along one wall, and an old rollback desk. Seated before the desk was a tall man with black hair and beard, reading out of a huge, worn volume. The door suddenly burst open, and a grimy, unshaven miner rushed into the room, gasping out, "Come quick, Doc, my partner's been shot." Within half an hour the doctor and his frantic companion were on their way over rutted, muddy roads in the open buggy drawn by a single horse, which the doctor used for all his transportation.

The year was 1878, the doctor, Henry Bergstein of Pioche, later director of the State Mental Hospital at Reno. At this time he had been practicing for six years in the state, with a territory that spread from Reno to Pioche, as well over halfway from Pioche to Las Vegas.

When he had first come to Nevada to practice in 1872, he had gone to the cemetery in Pioche to find just from reading the tombstones just what diseases he would probably have the greatest trouble treating. A walk through the cemetery revealed that of the 108 graves he found there, a total of three died a natural cause. As might have been expected, the majority of Dr. Bergstein's cases, as well as those handled by his colleagues, were gunshot wounds, knife slashes, and similar ailments of a rugged frontier life.

When Dr. Bergstein returned, after a three-day trip, from patching up his patient, a victim of an attempted claim-jumper, he found a letter from a Carson City friend, Dr. J.W. Waters. The letter contained an invitation to meet in Carson City on May 2 to help organize a state medical society of some sort.

Attending the meeting were seventeen practicing physicians from the western and southern part of the State, a small percentage of the 110 doctors registered in the State. The Nevada State Medical Association was formed as a result of that meeting. Chosen as its leaders were Dr. John W. Vanzant of Carson City, President; Dr. Waters, Vice-President; and Dr. A. Dawson, who with his stepbrother, Dr. H.H. Hogan, was one of the few practitioners in the then, small village of Reno, was elected secretary.

The doctors also established a uniform set of fees by which they all abided for several years. For a day call, the charge was $5; for a night call, $10; a normal confinement ran to $100, and surgery went from $100 up, depending on the nature of the operation and the ability of the patient to pay. The State Medical Association met more or less semi-annually for some years, but because of transportation difficulties interest gradually died, and the association became extinct.

By the time young Dr. W.H. Hood, fresh from medical school at the University of Michigan, arrived in Battle Mountain in 1886, interest had hit a new low. As he and other arrivals from the East began to take up practice in Nevada, however, they started a movement to revive the old medical association.

As a result to the renewed interest of the medical profession, they got a bill passed by the Nevada Legislature in 1887 that all births and deaths be recorded. Before this time no records of any kind had been kept. That some year, Dr. George H. Thomas, one of Nevada's outstanding doctors who had been practicing in Eureka and various other parts of the state since the close of the Civil War, moved his practice to Reno.

By 1894, the state association was back on its feet, although its members were still chiefly residents of Washoe, Ormsby and Storey counties. In 1899 the association achieved a major victory; a bill providing for establishment of a board of medical examiners and requiring that all practicing physicians be licensed was passed. This was the first real control placed on medical practitioners; before this, quacks of all sorts with fake medical diplomas flourished in the state.

On May 29, 1899, the first medical license in Nevada was given to Dr. Hood, who was still practicing in Battle Mountain. By this time the town of Reno had grown to a little city of 4,000. In 1901, when Dr. M.R. Walker decided to settle in Reno, there were eleven doctors already practicing. When Dr. Walker went to distribute his calling cards among the drug stores, he encountered one druggist, an old Englishman, who looked contemptuously at the card, then remarked, "Damn fool, too many doctors here now." For a short time it looked as though twelve doctors would be too many for the little town, but in the next two or three years it grew to support several more doctors. The next year Reno lost Dr. Hogan.

He was one of the first pioneers in the medical field to succeed. Among some of the newcomers to Reno in the next five years was Dr. Hood from Battle Mountain, who moved in 1904, after eighteen years of practice in the eastern part of the state. In the fall of that same year, a call went out to doctors of the state to meet December 19 for the purpose of reorganizing the now defunct medical association. Sixteen doctors attended the meeting and twenty-one, including Dr. Hood. Dr. Thoma, and Dr. Walker from Reno became founders of the new society. Chosen as officers were Dr. W.L. Moore, President, and Dr. J.L. Robinson, Secretary. Dr. Thoma was elected president in the following year. Exactly 1 month after this term expired on January 31, 1907, Dr. Thoma died. Nevada had lost one of its most beloved pioneer doctors, who had practiced 40 years in his beloved state. On May 25, 1907, Reno's doctors took another step toward cooperation within the profession. The Washoe County Medical Society was established with Dr. C.H. Hood as first president.

By 1910, the year Dr. Hood traded in his old buggy and prize team for a brand-new Lion 40, the main problem confronting Reno's doctors was the lack of hospitals. The forerunner of the present Saint Mary's Hospital on West 6th Street was started in 1907, but the facilities were not adequate for Reno's growing population. The hospital had grown out of an epidemic in 1907 of measles and scarlet fever. At that time, the Catholic nuns of Reno operated a boarding school on the southwest corner of 6th and Chestnut Streets. When the epidemic reached the school, the dormitory was converted into a hospital to house the infected children. When the epidemic had passed, sisters continued using the building as a hospital.

By 1912, the building, which at present serves as a convent was built as an addition to the hospital. The hospital provided facilities for many who would did not have a cure. In 1922, Saint Mary's Hosp. was listed as a Standard Hospital by the American College of Surgeons, the first of Reno hosp. to win that distinction.

Between 1910 and 1920, various private hospitals operated by physicians were opened, but none of these lasted. One the best known of these was the Mt. Rose Hospital, run by Dr. McKenzie until his death. During the 1920s the pressure for more hospitals continued, along with a need for more professionally trained nurses associated was established during this decade.

In 1930, Saint Mary's new building, the main part of the present structure was completed, containing 52 beds, modern laboratories and three modernized operating rooms.

In 1923, the county recognized the need for a public hospital providing hospitalization paid for according to the patient's ability to pay, promulgated a law providing for such a hospital. An old hospital had been organized in connection with the county poor farm some time before the turn of the century, but its equipment was outdated and unsatisfactory. It was not until 1932 that a satisfactory county hospital was built. The structure on Mill and Kirman streets, now known as the Washoe Medical Center, was erected. Since that time Veterans Hospital serving most of the veterans throughout the state, has been built.

In 1937, the east wing of Saint Mary's was added, furnishing as additional twenty-three beds and pharmacy. An addition to the rear of the wing was constructed in 1949, which provided facilities for 15 more patients. An addition under construction at the present time will be finished sometime this fall. It will provide 35 more beds, as well as a new kitchen, two new operating rooms, and an up-to-date maternity section.

The medical profession has made striking advances in the last seventy-five years. Its achievements are more dramatic and obvious than those made in other fields because medicine in Nevada was necessarily so primitive that modern miracles of science standout in sharp contrast. The members of the profession, although their organization, have agitated for such tremendous public projects as the building of Reno's sewage system, the establishment of an industrial insurance commission, organization of the Nevada State Nurses Association, establishment of a state board of health, and the construction well-equipped research laboratories.

The Washoe County Medical Society has at present [1951] eighty-four members, including highly trained general practitioners and specialists in 10 different fields, a far cry from that July day in 1901 when the gruff old druggist remarked that twelve doctors practicing in the city of Reno were too many.

EDITORS' NOTE:
- nsma was named the Nevada State Medical Society in 1878. We have chosen to

use nsma, the name when it was reformed in 1905. See the nsma in the Index for the initial founders and those involved in reforming the association.

- John La Rue Robinson was born in 1872 and received his MD from Keokuk Medical College in 1898. He was licensed in Reno in 1904 and was a leader in Nevada medicine for a number of years. Dr. Robinson organized Peoples Hospital and was president of nsma in 1923. He died in July 1950.

- In 2014, nsma is composed of 6 medical societies—Carson Douglas County, Central Counties, Clark County (formed in 1955), Elko County, Washoe County, and White Pine County.

NEVADA'S FIRST PEDIATRICIAN
DR. ANTHONY HUFFAKER

Anton P. Sohn MD

Dr. Anthony A. Huffaker was born in 1863 and graduated from Cooper Medical School in San Francisco. The school later became Stanford University School of Medicine. Huffaker came to Carson City in 1896. He is said to have been the first pediatrician in Nevada. Ten years later in 1907, Dr. Huffaker was elected president of nsma.

Dr. Huffaker decided in the early part of the 1900s that he should buy an automobile to use on his routine of daily visits to patients. He bought the car, studied his book of instructions, and boldly took it out on his rounds. Several hours later Mrs. Huffaker was in the front yard watering Dr. Huffaker's prize dahlias when the doctor came driving down the street. He called out to her but drove on past; in a few minutes he came back around the block, and with an agonized look on his face, he drove past again; the third time around he leaned out and called to his wife, "Go get the instruction book and throw it to me the next time around. I've forgotten how to stop the blamed machine!"

Vol. XVII, No. 2, Summer 2006

EDITORS' NOTE:

It is impossible to verify that Dr. Huffaker was the first pediatrician. In fact, many 19th-century women physicians only treated children and women; they could be considered pediatricians.

PUBLIC HEALTH IN NEVADA,
FIRST HUNDRED YEARS

Donald S. Kwalick MD

In March 1992 Nevada began its 100th year of 'organized' public health in the state. This report details the first one hundred years of public health in the rich history of our state.

THE FIRST FIFTY YEARS

The first Board of Health was composed of the governor and three appointed physicians—J.J. Henderson of Elko, J.A. Lewis of Reno, and S.L Lee of Carson City. Dr. Lee remained an active participant for twenty-three years.

Over this time, a great deal of energy was spent in development of vital statistics such as reporting of births, deaths, and disease. As late as 1900 Nevada did not require physicians to report "… all cases of contagious disease… and deaths from any cause."

In 1910, there were still no mandatory morbidity reports, although all counties (except Lander and Lincoln) were voluntarily making such reports. Finally, in March 1911, a state vital statistics statute was enacted, and in 1912, Nevada had its first morbidity and mortality statistics:

Disease	# Cases	# Deaths
Pneumonia	330	102
Pulmonary TB	190	52
Smallpox	215	3
Typhoid Fever	228	24

In 1913 state law required the Boards of County Commissioners to appoint local health officials at not less than $25 per month. All physicians were required to report all cases of smallpox, diphtheria, and scarlet fever within twenty-four hours, and all 'contagion' by the 5th of each month for the previous month. Willful neglect or refusal was subject to a fine of not less than $5 and no more than $25.

In 1920, Nevada was the only state without a full-time health officer, but in 1929, Nevada finally adopted the U.S. model vital statistics law and therefore for the first time, became part of the federal registration system for births and deaths. We were the last state in the Union to adopt this model law.

In 1934, forty years after establishing our Board of Health, Dr. John E. Worden became the first full-time State Health Officer. During the period from 1935 to 1940 the State Board of Health, with twenty-six full-time employees, was the state's fourth largest department. In the early 1940s the Board was reorganized into the Nevada State Department of Health, composed of eight divisions:

1. Administration and Training
2. Vital Statistics
3. Maternal and Child Health and
4. Crippled Children's Services
5. Dental Hygiene
6. Public Health Engineering
7. Local Health Administration, Epidemiology General Disease Control
8. Laboratories

During the first fifty years, the Health Department struggled to find qualified full-time staff. Development of an efficient system of reporting birth, death and disease statistics was one of the major problems. Only after the passage of state regulations for the reporting of communicable disease did Nevada finally join the rest of the nation with an effective Public Health law.

Vol. VIII, No. 1, Spring 1997

THE SECOND FIFTY YEARS

During the first fifty years, there were only four individuals who held the office of state health officer. The second fifty years of public health in Nevada, from 1942 until 1992, were times of enormous change in public health throughout the country. During the second half of the century there were twelve different state health officers, with two of them served for more than ten years. The position of state health officer was abolished by the Nevada Legislature in 1983 and reestablished in 1987. During this period Dr. George Reynolds served as acting state health officer.

In the early '40s and '50s, the Nevada Board of Health was composed of two physicians, one dentist, one layperson, and the governor. This board selected its chairman and the state health officer, who served as secretary to the board but was not a member. The state health officer also served as executive head of the Nevada Department of Health. It was a turbulent mixture of both public health and politics that formed the background for the current organization. These are some of the outstanding events that occurred during those second fifty years:

1947—A branch health laboratory established in Las Vegas.

1948—Dr. Daniel J. Hurley was appointed state health officer and provided stable leadership for 16 years. Physicians were appointed as county health officer in all Nevada counties.

1949—The Clark County Health Department was formed, and a full time health officer was appointed. Enabling legislation passed to receive Hill-Burton funding to build hospitals, nursing homes etc. Seven Hill-Burton projects were initiated.

1950—Sven of the seventeen counties have public health nursing services. Weekly news releases and radio programs regarding public health activities began.

1952—There was an unusual outbreak of Rocky Mountain Spotted Fever. Nevada suffered the worst polio epidemic, in its history, with 108 cases and 8 deaths. Hosp. surveys and inspections began.

1953—Reportable disease list was revised. New confidential reporting form adopted.

1954—Salk polio vaccinations began in Washoe County. Three fatal cases of botulism were reported.

1957—Special Children's Clinics established in Reno and Las Vegas. The Nevada Dental Society purchased a mobile unit for rural dental services.

1958—The Reno/Washoe County Health Department is organized.

1959—Food and drug laboratory activities transferred from University of Nevada to Nevada Department of Health (doh).

1960—Legislation enacted to provide care for indigent tuberculosis patients. doh reorganized into 6 bureaus: Environmental Health, Preventive Medical Services, Mental Health, Public Health Nursing, Hospital Services and Vital Statistics. Nevada Public Health Association established.

1962—Nevada has the highest birth rate in the U.S. Dr. John F. Carr resigns as Clark Co. health officer. District Health Department established in Clark Co. with financial responsibility.

1963—Dr. Otto Ravenholt appointed Clark County health officer. Nev. Health Depart. becomes the Division of Health.

1964—Bureau of Maternal and Child Health and Crippled Children's program began. Dr. Hurley replaced by Dr. W.T. Weathington and begins an era of rapid turnovers as health officer.

1966—Nevada is the first state in hew Region IX to have all participating hospitals certified for Medicare.

1967—Dr. William Bentley appointed to Nevada Board of Health. Rabies emergency in Ely and White Pine Counties.

1968—Deaths due to heart disease drop to below thirty percent for the first time in Nevada. Nevada is first state in the southwest U.S. to comply with Federal Clean Water Act.

1969—Division of Health bureaus centralized in Carson City except for laboratories and preventive medicine services. Infant death rate in Nevada is 3-5 points higher than U.S. average.

1970—In Washoe Co. Rubella becomes a reportable disease.

1972—Nevada becomes twenty-fourth state with Atomic Energy Commission (aec) agreement regulating radioactive material.

1973—Department of Health and Welfare becomes Department of Human Resources. Air/water pollution programs transferred to new Division of Environmental Protection under the Department of Conservation and Natural Resources. Bureau of Mental Health becomes Division of Mental Hygiene and Mental Retardation within Department of Human Resources. The Office of Emergency Medical Services is established.

1980—Improved pregnancy outcomes program started with federal funds, infant mortality rate falls markedly.

1981—State laboratory director, biostatistician, and medical director of community health services positions eliminated.

1983—State health officer, consumer health bureau chief positions eliminated.

1984—Federal Improved Pregnancy Outcome funds vanish. Infant mortality rate increases

1988—State health officer position reinstated. New positions created in Communicable Disease Control, aids prevention, Radiological Health, Long term care facility regulation, medical laboratory regulation. Two pediatricians hired for Special Children's Clinics.

1989—Health educator, laboratory director, biostatistician positions reinstituted. Nevada Legislature strengthens communicable disease statutes.

1990—State health officer, laboratory director and biostatistician positions filled.

1991-1992—Health planning transferred to Division of Health. Budget shortfalls necessitate twenty percent cuts.

1992—Cumulative aids cases exceed 1,000.

Vol. VIII, No. 2, Summer 1997

EDITORS' NOTE:

- Rocky Mountain Spotted Fever is caused by a group of bacteria named rickettsia that causes typhus and other febrile diseases. It grows inside of living cells—transmitted by ticks.

- According to Dr. Kwalick the 1980s began with budgetary problems. Despite a decade of shuffling positions, eliminating, and reinstitution of positions and turnover in leadership, the budgetary problems have persisted. Nevada continued to lead the nation in rates of lung cancer, deaths from trauma, liver cancer, low birth weight, and suicide. Dr. Kwalick, the State Health Officer until January 1997.

- Otto Ravenholt was born in 1927 in Wisconsin and graduated from the University of Minnesota School of Medicine in 1958. He served in the U.S. Army from 1947 to 1952 and obtained his MS in public health in 1960. After working three years in Topeka, Kansas, he came to Nevada in 1964. Under Governor Robert Laxalt he served as director of the Nevada Department of Health and Human Services. Dr. Ravenholt has also served as administrator of Southern Nevada Memorial Hospital and the Clark County Coroner's office. He was director of the Clark County Health Department for 36 years before he retired in 1999.

- Daniel Hurley was born in Idaho in 1902 graduated in medicine from Creighton University, and received a master's degree in public health from Harvard. In 1928, he practiced in Eureka, Nevada, where he remained until World War II when he joined the U.S. Navy Reserve. In 1948 he moved to Carson City and became the state health officer. He died in 1973.

NEVADA'S FIRST FULL-TIME HEALTH OFFICER
Dr. John Worden

Anton P. Sohn MD

The law creating the Nevada State Board of Health was enacted in 1893, and a number of physicians were appointed to the board. They were all part-time health officers. According to Dr. Don Kwalick, Dr. John Edward Worden was the first full-time officer. John was born in Canada in February 1875. On June 15, 1889, he graduated from Northwestern Medical School, and by 1892, he was living in Milwaukee. Dr. Worden studied public health at the University of Michigan and was licensed in 1908 in Fallon where he was Churchill County Health Officer.

In 1916, he moved to Elko and was appointed its county health officer. In 1936, Governor Richard Kirman appointed Dr. Worden to be the 1st full-time State Health Officer with the princely salary of $2,500. Governor Kirman asked for his resignation two times in 1938 because Worden ran for the U.S. Senate, and Kirman felt this was a conflict of interest. Worden refused both times, but in 1939 he resigned after a severe injury resulting from an auto accident. That year he moved to San Francisco to live with his daughter. He died there in 1959. His obituary in the December 29, 1959, *Reno Evening Gazette*, includes a picture of him and states that he had two children.

EDITORS' NOTE:

This research was undertaken when Dr. Trudy Larson, the UNRSOM Public Health Program Director, asked for the name of the first state health officer in Nevada in order to honor him by awarding student scholarships in his name. I asked Guy Rocha for his help. "Dr. John Worden, without question, deserves the honor for his thirty one years of public health service to Nevada."

Vol. XXII, No. 3, Fall 2011

MIDWIVES IN EARLY NEVADA

Phyllis Cudek, Historian

The wagon trains bearing pioneers included pregnant women and midwives who could attend to them during childbirth. Isolated communities through which the wagon trains passed also had a need for the knowledge and experience brought by midwives. Outbreaks of smallpox, influenza, and other such illnesses required as much medical assistance as could be found in the area, and midwives were often the only persons available with any medical experience.

Their knowledge of home remedies and use of herbal ingredients was often invaluable to the settlers' health. So scarce were medical supplies that cactus fiber was occasionally used to suture wounds.

Although the importance of midwives was undeniable, they rarely listed themselves as 'professionals' in county census reports or city directories. For example, in *Bishop's Directory of Virginia City, Gold Hill, Silver City, Carson City, and Reno, 1878-79*, professions such as dressmakers, milliners, domestics, teachers, and ladies' nurses were listed; however, only two midwives, Mrs. Julia Bellmerre of Virginia City and Mrs. S.M. Drannan of Reno, were acknowledged in addition to Mrs. Helen Anderson of Reno, who was listed as midwife and physician. Midwives were crucial to the sustained population growth of rural communities. They enabled the West to grow and prosper because of their maternal and childbirth skills.

The Church of Latter Day Saints contributed widely to the presence and importance of midwifery in Nevada in the 19th- and early 20th-centuries. Settlements established under the direction of the Mormon Church took families to remote areas of the state. The proliferation of children demonstrated the need for childbirth assistance; therefore, women were often chosen from their communities to travel to Salt Lake City to be trained in the techniques of midwifery and who then would return to their communities to practice.

In 1891, Panaca in southeastern Nevada was such a community. One of its midwives was Mariah Berdilla Rich (nee Atchison). This woman delivered Nevada W. Driggs, who later wrote an article for the *Nevada Historical Quarterly* describing childbirth in a small western town. Two other women from the Mormon Church, well known in their community of White Pine Country were Mrs. Mary Leicht Oxborrow and Mrs. Margaret Christina Arnoldus Windous.

Author Effie Oxborrow Read writes about midwives, Mary Leich Oxborrow (grandmother) and Margaret Christina Arnoldus Windous, in White Pine County.

A True History of White Pine County, Nevada. In 1900, Mrs. Mary Leicht Oxborrow came from St. George, Utah. She had been set aside by the Church authorities as a midwife and doctor for the community of Lund. She already had sons and daughters there. Her excellence as a Doctor cannot be over-commended. She made her own medicines, salves, face cream, and had keen knowledge of herbs. She accomplished tremendous medical feats in care of broken bones and cuts. She delivered 235 babies, two of whom were her own great grandchildren. She was an excellent musician and was a beloved character.

Effie Read continues later in her book with information on another much-admired midwife and doctor, Margaret Christine Arnoldus Windous: In 1908 the Latter Day Saints Church requested that each ward of the Church send at least one Relief Society member to Salt Lake City to train under the direction of Dr. Ramona B. Pratt. Mrs. Windous had 8 children and limited education, but she accomplished this mission and received certification for practicing obstetrics and nursing. She was the 'country doctor,' and it was necessary for her to make many lonely trips across the desert in the dead of night with her little black buggy and faithful horse, Dolly.

Mrs. Windous lived in Nevada from 1899, had a Maternity Home in Lund, and delivered more than 1,000 babies. "Her patients were of all nationalities and religions," writes Read. Most communities had their own midwife who could be summoned for an expected birth. Midwives, unlike physicians, gave family assistance in ways other than delivering a child. A midwife would leave her own family while she gave physical and emotional support to the expectant woman, often cooking meals, doing laundry, housecleaning, and caring for other family members after the birth of a new baby. This service would often last several days before and/or after the childbirth; frontier women helped women in any way possible.

In Nevada's early days it was not unusual for a mother to be a midwife to her daughter, daughter-in-law, her granddaughter, or for a sister to be a midwife to her own sister. Although a midwife was usually a woman who had given birth to children herself, it was not uncommon for a young girl to assist a family member in the birthing process.

A few illustrations of midwifery activities follow. Anna Mueller Engel Neddenriep was a qualified midwife who wore a long black cape as a symbol of her profession. Her Carson Valley neighbors often referred her to as an angel of mercy.

Around 1900, Mrs. Mary 'Granny' Dakin offered hospital services in Elko after having been a midwife for many years and also having taught midwifery to her daughter, Mrs. Tillie Roach. Mrs. Bill Bradley, a midwife for the White Pine County area was 'untutored,' but would, "Often…. tie her own small baby to her back Indian-style, saddle a pony, and ride twenty miles or more to be on hand for the blessed event." Mrs. Scott from Osceola was midwife for Anna Day Swallow in the Shoshone area around the 1880s.

Despite her lack of formal medical training 'Little Mrs. Dr. Swallow' cared for burns, pneumonia, and delivered babies. She would often travel in the dead of night by horse and sleigh in two feet of snow to reach a patient. The treatment given by midwives was usually non-interventionist. Although forceps had been used for hundreds of years, and were sometimes present in the 'medical bag' of a midwife, they were often reserved for use by a physician for a difficult delivery. Administration of ergot, a commercially prepared medicine formulated from a rye grain fungus, was used by midwives and physicians to produce contractions of the uterus and curtail postpartum bleeding.

Other home remedies known by particular midwives were no doubt used to provide comfort, but generally childbirth was on the frontier without aid or medication.

Puerperal fever, commonly known as childbed fever, was a constant threat to the life of a delivering mother. However, once the importance of cleanliness and sterilization became known, this condition became less prevalent. As Nevada's population grew, some of the larger communities such as Elko, Ely, and Reno had maternity homes or hospitals, which were usually operated by nurses or midwives. Some women would come for the birth of a child and then remain for several days to heal and regain strength before returning home to their families.

Because of the anonymity of many midwives in Nevada's wide-open spaces, finding and documenting names of women who aided other women, and also performed medical services for their communities, is difficult and many times impossible. Terminology in reference to midwives adds frustration to research efforts; midwives may also be referred to as ladies' nurses—Midwives included Doctresses, which could also refer to female physicians, or merely those who treat sick or injured people. Also present were a few men who signed birth certificates as '*accoucheur*,' which can be interpreted as male midwife or an obstetrician, but not necessarily a physician. The moral atmosphere of the 1800s and early 1900s contributed to the obscurity of midwife identification in that 'genteel' women did not discuss birthing nor intimate personal life in general. By 1900, births in the United States were assisted approximately equally by both midwives and physicians. This was not true in the sparsely populated state of Nevada.

Vol. VIII, No. 4, Winter 1997-8

NEVADA'S FIRST PATHOLOGIST
DR. OSCAR JOHNSTONE

Anton P. Sohn MD

Born in Iowa in 1871, Dr. Oscar Percy Johnstone graduated from Chicago's Rush Medical College in 1905. He instructed at Columbia University, practiced a short time in Pittsburgh, and was an instructor at the Denver College of Medicine before he came to Reno to be one of Nevada's first pathologists, if not the first. He was in charge of the State Hygienic Laboratory, but he resigned after five years to associate with Dr. W.L. Samuels in a clinic at the Masonic Temple.

At 1:00 pm on November 9, 1916, Dr. Johnstone was found dead sitting in his office chair. An office attendant, Miss Ada Hussman, had noticed him two hours earlier sitting in the exact same position and thought him to be asleep. Doctors S.K. Morrison and Mullins did the autopsy and assigned the cause of death to be atheromatous degeneration of the arteries of the heart. Johnstone was considered to be one of the leading authorities "…on the West Coast in bacteriology and pathological diagnosis." (NSJ, November 10, 1916) He was a member of the Nevada State Board of Health and was vice-president of wcms.

Two weeks after Dr. Johnstone's death his widow, Bertha Shryock Johnstone, administered chloroform to kill herself and their three children, Eric, six years, Thorwald, four years, and William, less than six months. Eric and William survived but on November 26, Bertha and Thorwald died. They were buried next to Dr. Johnstone in Mountain View Cemetery.

Vol. XXII, No. 2, Summer 2011

EDITORS NOTE:

Dr. Oscar Percy Johnstone was born in Missouri in 1871. He graduated from Rush Medical College in Chicago in 1905, and later that year was appointed professor of pathology at the Colorado School of Medicine in Boulder. He practiced in Pittsburgh, being licensed in Reno in 1911.

Johnstone was associated with the State Hygienic Laboratory as a pathologist and bacteriologist.

Dr. Mark F. Boyd, Nevada's second pathologist, graduated from the University of Iowa Medical College in 1911 and was licensed in Nevada in 1914 and noted to be a pathologist.

WASHOE COUNTY MEDICAL SOCIETY
The Beginning
Minutes of the First Meeting

Reno, Nevada May 25, 1907

The Washoe County (Nevada) Medical Society was duly organized on this date by the following named Physicians: C.H. Woods, John Lewis, M.R. Walker, L. J. Richie, B.F. Cunningham, C.H. Francis, Barrett D. Bice, R. St. Clair C.E. Masson, W.H. Hood, S.M. Morrison, R. L. Rice, J.L. Robinson, Kistler, [Gilmour] Roberts, R.M.W. O'Neal. .

On motion duly made, seconded and carried Dr. Woods was elected temporary president, Dr. John Lewis temporary vice-president, and Dr. C.E. Masson temporary Secretary. It was moved, seconded and carried that the temporary officers be elected permanent officers.

Dr. Cunningham moves that a Committee on By-Laws consisting of three members be appointed by the chair. Motion seconded and carried The President appointed the following: Dr. Cunningham, Dr. Morrison and Dr. Walker. Dr. Hood moves that the Board of Censors, consisting of three members be appointed by the chair. Motion Seconded and carried. The President appointed the following: Dr. Hood, Dr. Kistler and Dr. Francis.

Owing to the intended departure from the State of our newly elected President, Dr. Morrison moves, seconded by Dr. St. Clair that the following resolution be adopted and a copy be presented to Dr. Woods: Resolved: that the Secretary of the Washoe Co. Medical Society be and he is hereby instructed to furnish our departing President, Dr. Woods with a letter of introduction to the San Diego Co. (California) Medical Society in taken of the esteem which he is held by the members of this Society—Motion was carried unanimously. Addresses were then made by a number of the members of this Society and after a vote of thanks to the Elks for their courtesy in loaning their rooms to the

Society, the meeting adjourned subject to the call of the chair.

Signed, Chas. E. Masson, Secretary

Vol. VIII, No. 2, Summer 1997

FIRST KNOWN AUTOPSY IN NEVADA
Dr. Anton Tjader

Violence was no stranger in Nevada, and in fact, the first legal execution occurred in Carson City on November 30, 1860, when Nevada was part of the Utah Territory.

Bernard Cherry who lived in Carson City was shot and killed near Dr. King's house in Carson City by Jonathan Carr, a former Pony Express rider and outlaw who robbed emigrants on their way to California. After the murder Carr fled to California where he was captured in Tuolumne County.

Carr confessed to the crime and was tried and hanged near the residence of Dr. Benjamin L King where the crime had been committed. Doctors George Munckton and Charles Daggett pronounced Carr dead, and Dr. Anton Tjader did the autopsy. For his efforts Tjader was paid $50, which was equivalent to two weeks salary for a doctor.

Vol. I, No. 4, Winter 1990-91

NEVADA'S MALPRACTICE CRISIS

Tom Brady MD

Practicing medicine in Nevada over the last several years has been complicated by medical professional liability issues. Perhaps one of the most serious adverse effects of malpractice, from a doctor's point of view, is its impact on the physician-patient relationship. It is essential that an open, trusting, caring, and aggressive doctor-patient relationship exist for the best medical care. If physicians see patients as potential adversaries, medical care clearly will suffer. We have always been patient advocates–not their adversaries.

During the period 1935 to 1975, eighty percent of all malpractice lawsuits were filed in the last five years of that period. Amounts awarded to plaintiffs were going up because of the influence of inflation, increasingly liberal judges and juries, and aggressive trial lawyers. From 1974 to 1976, under-prepared and under-funded professional liability carriers or insurance companies left the market and a crisis of availability of insurance developed. Some physicians went bare and had no insurance.

To help solve the problem, Nevada created a physician-owned, non-profit insurance company, Nevada Medical Liability Insurance Company (nmlic). About the same time, the Doctors Company was created in California. This relieved the availability of insurance problem.

Nevada had ventured into voluntary medical-legal screening panels in the 1960s. The idea was to keep frivolous lawsuits from going to court and provide quicker settlements where there has been malpractice and injury occurred. Hopefully, this would also lower costs. In 1975 the Nevada Legislature made these voluntary panels mandatory for all claims. The panels were less than satisfactory; however, thirty percent of claims rejected by the panels went to court anyway. There were so many claims that the panels were terribly backlogged, and the plaintiffs' attorneys used the panel as a means of discovery using the accumulated information in subsequent litigation. As frustration with the panels increased, the trial lawyers, insurance companies, and doctors all joined in lobbying the legislature to again make this medical-legal screening panel voluntary and this passed in 1981.

Costs for liability insurance continued to soar. Malpractice insurance premiums increased on average of twenty-two percent per year from 1980 to 1985. Multi-million-dollar judgments became more common in areas such as neonatal pediatrics, neurosurgery, and especially obstetrics. The coverage available was $1 million per case and $3 million total for three cases. Since almost all the babies delivered in rural Nevada were delivered by family practitioners, they simply could not afford the $36,000 per year cost of insurance and stopped delivering pregnant women. Obstetrics in rural Nevada was gone. A new crisis had developed.

In 1985, the Nevada State Medical Association began a long and ultimately successful lobbying effort for tort Reform. The Nevada Trial Lawyers Association (ntla) opposed this effort. The four basic tort Reforms proposed were:

1. Limits on liability (cap on non-economic loss)
2. Periodic payments of court awards (In lieu of lump sum pay)
3. Limitation of attorney contingency fees (sliding-scale increments)
4. Collateral source payments (prevention of double payments in court awards)

I was involved in the lobbying effort, and there were many intense discussions with the trial lawyers and legislators. Finally, a deadlocked legislature and the Judiciary Committee led by Attorney Bob Sader directed us to meet and make a compromise proposal. Attorneys Bill Bradley and David Gamble, Dr. Anton Sohn, and I met, and the outcome was a new medical-legal screening panel. The new panel was much more effective.

1. It was mandatory.
2. It was based on records only (the plaintiff and defendant did not have to sit and face each other).
3. The results were admissible in court.
4. If the panel found for the defendant and the claimant does not win in court, the defendant must be awarded costs and attorney fees.
5. If the panel finds for the plaintiff, a settlement conference must be held.

The new medical-legal screening panel proved to be successful, but the battle for real tort Reform was just started. The issue of medical malpractice would not go away despite the success of the screening panel. Medical liability created tension between the professions of law and medicine.

Physicians believe that reform of the tort system is needed because the present system is too slow, too expensive, unfair and doesn't consider the life and death decisions that doctors face and make and confront daily. They believe that a system, which gives an average of thirty to forty cents per dollar awarded to injured patients is not effective.

Lawyers, on the other hand, see the tort system as a fundamental part of our social system, which rights civil wrongs and holds doctors accountable. They see themselves as instruments of as such, the face-off has stood.

It would not end until 2004 when true tort Reform was passed through the initiative process on the public ballot and then enacted by the legislature.

EDITORS' NOTE:

- In the summer of 2002, Governor Kenny Guinn convened a special session of the legislature solely to consider and adopt additional reforms. These included a $350,000 cap on noneconomic damages except in cases involving exceptional circumstances. The special session also repealed the mandatory screening panel that many physicians wish was still in effect. In 2004 an initiative was placed on the ballot in a general election, which abolished any exception to the $350,000 damage cap on noneconomic damages. It was passed overwhelming by the voters and became law.

- tort (Latin *torquere* 'to twist') is defined as a wrongful act or an infringement of a right (other than under contract) leading to civil legal liability.

- When Nevada's malpractice crisis came to a head in the 1970s and '80s, many doctors in Nevada went 'bare,' which means they did not buy malpractice insurance in order to avoid the huge cost of the premium. During that time the average malpractice lawsuit cost to defend, even if the case was frivolous, $50,000. Furthermore, there was little protection legally from such a suit being filed. As a result, many insurance companies settled the case and did not go to court.

- In the mid-1975, the *Wall Street Journal* got word of Nevada doctors going 'bare' and ran an article on the crisis. In July 1975 Rick Pugh, nsma ceo, got a call from the producers of cbs' *60 Minutes* asking to do a segment on the escalating malpractice insurance crisis in Nevada.

Dr. Jack Talsma, president of wcms agreed to meet with cbs producer Sheldon Gordon to work out details. Pugh recalls making reservations at Eugene's restaurant for him and wife Charlotte, Jack and wife Sydney, and Sheldon Gordon. At dinner, plans were made to meet with reporter Morley Safer in wmc Administrator Carroll Ogren's office the following week. Reporter Mike Wallace was designated to do the interview, but due to a scheduling conflict, Morley Safer got the assignment. Ultimately, going 'bare" was not a good strategy and some doctors got sued for frivolous reasons and paid the settlement amount out of their practice income. Needless to say, this brought a halt to going 'bare.'

CHAPTER III:
NATIVE AMERICAN MEDICINE

North American Natives were probably better off—health wise—before Europeans invaded their country. Life was harsh in the Great Basin and starvation a threat during the harsh, cold winters, but the inhabitants were free of the many diseases that killed thousands in Europe, Africa, and Asia. The list is long and includes smallpox, tuberculosis, malaria, venereal disease, and numerous other contagious diseases. This article will deal with how Indigenous Americans treated native diseases and diseases brought into this country.

Nine tribal groups roamed the Great Basin, and each had its unique practices when dealing with illness. The nine groups anthropologists recognize in the Intermountain West are Western Shoshone, Northern Shoshone/Bannock, Eastern Shoshone, Ute, Southern Paiute, Kawaiisu, Owens Valley Paiute, Northern Paiute and Washoe. Although these nine groups had distinct and separate practices, they dealt with disease in a similar fashion. They not only respected each other's practices, but they borrowed from each other.

The Native American health system dealt with health, disease, mental illness, and rites of passage—birth, naming, puberty, and old age. Various individuals in the tribe had their place in this coordinated and coherent system that had a rich, strongly conservative tradition. The women of the tribe oversaw menstrual rites and the birth process. On occasion a shaman might be called during a difficult birth. The men were concerned with hunting and the passage of young men into the warrior class. On a more profound level, medicine men accompanied the war parties for religious and medical needs.

The treatment of diseases by American Indians was a complex combination of medicine and religion. A healthy individual had a harmonious relationship with the supernatural, while disease was a disturbance of this balance. Healing, brought about in one of several manners, reestablished the balance. In the Great Basin there were three classes of health providers—the herbalist, the medicine man, and the shaman.

The herbalist treated minor ailments such as broken bones, minor trauma, indigestion, etc. He or she mixed concoctions and had knowledge of plants and herbs. In some tribes they practiced bloodletting. On another level was the medicine man, who had 'power' in his curing activities, but his powers were considerably less than the shaman, who healed in deep trances and went on soul journeys to rescue the soul of his patient. Modern medicine would recognize the shaman as a psychotherapist. All of the Great Basin tribal groups used these healers in a similar manner, but there were subtle differences, as the following essays will reveal.

GREAT BASIN
NATIVE AMERICAN HERBAL MEDICINE

Janet K. Holmes, UNR History Student

Fifty-two plants are said to constitute medicine for 'colds,' fifty-seven for venereal diseases (with an occasional distinction between gonorrhea and syphilis), forty-four for 'swelling,' thirty-four for diarrhea, thirty-seven for 'rheumatism,' and forty-eight for various stomach indispositions including 'stomachache.'

These herbs and plants played an important role in healing. Data indicates that the Paiute were highly sophisticated botanists. Beyond the Paiute, the Shoshone were probably the most advanced tribe in terms of medicinal plant lore. For the Goshute, it appears that all members of the tribe had some working knowledge of the medicinal herbs. The Washoe were considered to have the least plant lore and borrowed from neighboring tribes. The Shoshone and Paiute were known to have traded medicinal plants outside of the Great Basin. Unlike the Washoe people they also traveled across the Great Basin to seek medicinal plants. This would account for their differences in knowledge of medicinal botany.

Because of the hundreds of varieties of plants used within their ethno-botanical medicine, it is not possible, within this venue, to cover every plant that the Great Basin people used for herbal cure or to cover the traditional preparation of each remedy. Therefore, we will briefly examine only approximately fifty species of plants and their uses. The list is alphabetically listed by common English plant names, but we will be glad to supply the scientific botanical name for those who are interested.

It is recognized that Native Americans used many plants that were pharmacologically active, such as ephedra, and were used appropriately. It is also know that, as a rule, Great Basin Native Americans did not suffer from scurvy because many of the plants were dried and used during periods when fresh plants were not available. Consequently, Vitamin C was ingested from these dried leafy plants.

Alumroot was used to make a tonic for use in general debility, as well as for heart trouble, venereal disease, high fevers, eyewash, liver problems, and diarrhea. In addition, it was used as an astringent and as a treatment for colic.

Arrow Weed was used for bloody diarrhea, and indigestion.

Balsamroot was used for severe stomach problems as well as bladder troubles

Biscuit root, Toza, Cough Root, Fern-Leaf or Carrot-Leaf was employed to treat trachoma, swellings, sprains, sore throat, gonorrhea, hay fever, colds, coughs, bronchitis, fevers, chest congestion, influenza, pneumonia, and as an antiseptic for small pox, rashes, sores and cuts. Biscuit root was also considered a curative for tuberculosis. It is still commonly used to treat arthritis, colds, and influenza.

Black Cottonwood was used for headaches, venereal diseases, tuberculosis, stomach disorders and general disability (blood tonic).

Brass Buttons was used for constipation, stomachaches, and cramps. It also acted as an emetic, physic, and eyewash.

Bristlecone Pine was used to draw out boils and was used to minister to sores.

Butterball was used as a cold medicine. It was also an eye medicine, and a remedy for stomachaches, and venereal diseases.

Button Snakewood was used for diarrhea.

California Incense Cedar was considered to protect against contagious diseases.

Cow Parsnip was used for toothaches, sore throats, coughs, colds, diarrhea, tuberculosis, rheumatism, and to benefit healing of wounds.

Creosote Bush was believed to be a general cure-all. It had analgesic and antiseptic properties. It was used to stimulate urination, to cure venereal diseases, colds, rheumatism, chicken pox, burns, and bowel cramps, and to aid in new skin formation. It worked as a styptic and, in recent years, it has been useful for treating cancer [It was also called Greasewood because of its extensive medicinal use. *Greasewood Tablettes* bulletin is named after the bush.]

Dodder was believed to induce sterility.

Ephedra, Mormon Tea, Indian Tea, or Squaw tea was used as a treatment for venereal diseases like syphilis and gonorrhea. It was also used for ailments of the kidneys and cramps. It was also used for bladder disorders, colds, blood purifier, circulation, delayed or difficult menstruation, and stomach disorders. When combined with other plants, it treated diarrhea, cure for sores, and burns. Some considered it to be a curative for backaches and anemia.

False Hellebore or Skunk Cabbage was used as a contraceptive. In addition, it was used for venereal diseases, sore throats, heavy colds, inflamed tonsils, swellings, rheumatism, sore nipples, infections, sores, cuts, boils, blood poisoning, and as a liniment. It was applied to snake bites, burns, bruises, toothaches, and fevers.

Gourd was used for venereal diseases (gonorrhea and syphilis) as well as an emetic and physic. It was a remedy for bloating and for worms. Gourd plants were also considered to be a cure-all by some indigenous people.

Horehound was believed to stimulate blood circulation. It also acted as a cough, cold, and respiratory aid.

Horsetail Rush was taken for kidney problems. It was used as diuretic, eyewash, and for urinary tract infections.

Jimson Weed was not used for medicinal purposes. However, it was known for its narcotic properties. It was used on occasion to render a person unconscious.

Juniper was used as a blood tonic, treating venereal disease, headaches, colds, disinfectant, fever, measles, burns, and wounds.

Lovage was made into a cough treatment.

Manzanita was used for venereal disease. In addition, manzanita was used for poison oak, and wounds.

Mint, Spearmint or Peppermint was used in a large variety of afflictions like colic, stomachaches, indigestion, diarrhea, headaches, colds, fevers, sore throats, and to reduce swelling. It was also used for heart problems. Spearmint leaves cured an upset stomach; and treated cough. Peppermint was used for gas pains.

Milkweed was employed for headaches and ringworm. It also could have drawn out snakebite poison.

Pink Sand was applied to burns.

Prince's Plume, Desert Plume, or Indian Cabbage was used to treat sore gums and teeth, earaches, rheumatic pains, and general weakness after an illness. It was used during a diphtheria epidemic to relieve pain and congestion of the throat.

Puffball was considered beneficial for swellings and sores.

Quaking Aspen was used for venereal diseases. Some indigenous people insisted that this had no medicinal value.

Rabbitbrush was made into remedies for colds, stomach disorders, and bloody diarrhea. It was also rubbed into the scalp to stimulate freer breathing. A general tonic was also made out of this. A liniment came from rabbitbrush as well.

Sagebrush was used as a headache remedy and used for rheumatism. Sagebrush was also used in healing ceremonies. Old black leaves were used on baby rashes.

Sandwort was used as eyewash.

Serviceberry was used for snow blindness.

Single-Leaf Pinion was frequently mixed with other plants and used for colds, venereal diseases, rheumatism, tuberculosis, fevers, nausea, chronic indigestion, influenza, pneumonia, bowel trouble, diarrhea, kidney problems, small pox, ruptures, sciatic pains, chest congestion, and as part of a post-childbirth tonic. It was used as a treatment for insect bites, swellings, sores, rashes, and cuts, or for drawing out boils and slivers. In addition, it was a sore throat remedy, intestinal parasites, worms, and muscular soreness.

Smokebush was used as a cough and cold remedy, as well as used to treat pneumonia, tuberculosis, influenza, whooping cough, stomachaches, toothaches, small pox, measles, venereal diseases, muscular pains, diarrhea, sores, rheumatism, face neuralgia, incontinence, kidney trouble or to induce urination.

Snowberry or Waxberry: was used for stomach pains and indigestion. These plants also helped to relieve the pains of childbirth.

St. John's Wort was used for bullet wounds, cuts, swellings, aching feet, toothaches, and venereal diseases.

Sulphur Flower was used for rheumatism, lameness, stomachaches, and colds.

Tobacco was employed to expel worms, as well as treat athlete's foot, asthma, tuberculosis, swellings, rheumatism, cuts, sores, snakebites, hives, eczema, skin infections or irritations. Tobacco was also used for decayed tooth pain. It also functioned as a cold remedy. It functioned as a physic and an emetic. It was used in the healing ritual.

Violet was considered to be a sweat inducer. Canadian Violets were used for lung trouble.

White Fir was believed to cure tuberculosis, venereal diseases, sores, boils, cuts, and lung troubles.

White-Sage or Winterfat was used as an anti-lice treatment, as well as a general scalp and hair tonic. It was believed to hold anti-graying and anti-baldness properties, as well as a potential hair-restorer. It was also used to relieve eye soreness. This helped to alleviate intermittent fevers. It aided in relieving respiratory ailments.

White Sand was employed for swellings.

Wild Buckwheat was used for tuberculosis, cough, lameness, rheumatism, and bladder trouble.

Wild Geraniums were used for upset-stomach, swollen feet, venereal diseases, sore eyes, ulcers, and colds and as a contraceptive.

Wild Mustard was used on burns.

Wild Rose or Woods' Rose was used for cuts, sores, wounds, intestinal influenza, bloody diarrhea, burns, swellings, boils, and as a general tonic or physic. It also was a cold remedy.

Yarrow had a wide range of medicinal uses e.g. a liniment for muscular pain, an itch remedy, stomachaches, indigestion, swellings, sores, rashes, fevers, headaches, sore eyes, colic, dyspepsia, kidney problems, local anesthetic, post-childbirth blood tonic, bladder ailments. It was also used for toothaches and gas pains. It was also used for colds, and bruises.

Yellow Dock, Indian Rhubarb, or Curly Dock is considered to be a common weed across the Great Basin.

Depending on the preparation, it was used to treat rheumatic swellings, bruises, burns, liver disorder and venereal diseases. It was also used as a pain reliever, a blood purifier, cure for diarrhea, and as a general tonic. In addition, it was used for a variety of ailments (e.g. scurvy, scales, running sores, skin eruptions, and itch reliever). It was used to treat stomachaches. (It was also smoked in ceremonies.)

Yucca, Spanish Bayonet, or Lord's Candle was used for blindness and skin irritation.

SUMMARY

Many of these herbs were also used for veterinary purposes. Beyond botanical remedies, there were many non-plant remedies that were also used by the Great Basin People as well. These included such treatments as using breast milk for a nursing baby's sore eyes, skunk grease on chapped skin, and horse urine for broken and itching pustules. In addition, the fat from some animal hearts was thought to be a cure for tuberculosis.

Within this paper, we have only begun to glimpse the extensive medicinal knowledge used by the Great Basin indigenous people. It is clear to see that these Great Basin people were creative in their cures. One can tell by the wide variety of plants for certain diseases (e.g. venereal diseases and rheumatism) that they had difficulty in finding reliable remedies. This seemed to be especially true for ailments that were brought in through European contact. It was also well known that various cures were adapted from their immigrant neighbors, and they, in turn, borrowed from the Native Americans.

By looking at these curatives, one can also gain perspective about the kinds of maladies that were most common. The indigenous Great Basin people found a wealth of medicinal riches amongst what would be considered to be to be mostly a wasteland of worthless desert by many modern Americans. It is hoped that modern Great Basin inhabitants, as well as Americans in general, may benefit from a better understanding of the knowledge and gain a true appreciation of these old aboriginal ways.

Vol. XVI, No. 1, Spring 2005,

Vol. XVI, No. 2, Summer 2005

NEVADA'S NATIVE AMERICAN HEALERS

Anton P. Sohn MD

SHOSHONE

The Western Shoshone occupied the largest territory extending from the depths of arid Death Valley and adjacent Panamint Mountains north to the Idaho border and east to include the Great Salt Lake. Most of this area was sparsely inhabited and, in fact, was the last area in the United States where settlers and the Army displaced the resident Native Americans. Forts Halleck and Ruby were located in the western half of the Western Shoshone land.

The Western Shoshone practiced medicine on two levels—curing supernatural disease by the shaman and treating other disease by the herbalist. Most injury and common minor illness were not considered to be caused by a supernatural phenomenon and were treated with herbs and home remedies similar to folk medicine as it was practiced by non-native settlers. To accomplish this task, various members of the tribe gathered the plants during the appropriate seasons, dried them and pulverized them for later use.

Several plants used in modern pharmacology (for example, ephedra, known as ephedrine) were used by Great Basin Indians. Of all the Native American groups in the Great Basin, the Western Shoshone had the greatest knowledge of plants and their medicinal uses. Furthermore, they carefully guarded their identification. In contrast, the Washoe had little knowledge of herbs and traded for them with neighboring California tribes.

Most serious illnesses in the Western Shoshone required treatment by a medicine man. Some medicine men healed in a light trance while others became more deeply entranced. Only in a deep trance could the shaman leave his body, become ecstatic, and rescue the soul of the sick person who was usually suffering from a disease with altered consciousness such as a coma or delirium.

The shaman was either a generalist with general curing ability or a specialist who was known to cure a specific disease such as a rattlesnake bite. This power was usually acquired in a dream in which the shaman saw himself curing a patient with a specific problem.

Central to medical practice of the shaman was the concept that disease was caused by the intrusion of an object within the body. The Shoshone believed that an arrow-shooting dwarf caused disease. Therefore, the shaman healed by sucking out a foreign object such as a stick or blood and displaying the object for all to see.

Each shaman in the Western Shoshone tribe practiced the sucking or healing ritual in his distinct and unique manner. In one healing ritual the shaman piled sagebrush around a fire pit and placed the sick person on a pile of sage. The shaman sang and meditated, and then placed his mouth on the diseased area and sucked out the pain. If the illness was more serious the shaman gave a longer treatment with chanting and singing, fasting, making sacrifices, and more important, he used sacred eagle feathers. In another healing ceremony the Native American doctor drew lines with a sacred (diatomaceous) rock on his patient and instructed the patient to go to the river the next day to sprinkle water, pray, and make a sacrifice.

In leaving the body disease could be due to a transgression of the soul. Laying on of hands was also an important part of the ritual. This practice is similar to the Christian practice of healing by laying on of hands, an important psychological factor in healing.

The Western Shoshone also believed that evil medicine doctors or sorcerers practiced witchcraft and caused disease. A shaman who refused to treat a patient or who failed to invoke a cure was considered evil. In the event that a healing ceremony did not produce a cure, the fee was returned. On a much more serious level there was an unwritten law that if a shaman lost three patients he should die—malpractice punishment at its extreme.

At Fort Ruby, a shaman lost his third patient and members of the Shoshone tribe decided to kill him. Mr. Wines, a pioneer 19th-century rancher who was trusted, called them together and informed them that he would send for the soldiers if they murdered the shaman. The Shoshones returned to their wikiups with a guarantee from the shaman that he would give up medicine practice.

In addition to shamanism and herbs, the Western Shoshone believed in hydrotherapy. Since ancient times, they used water from Medicine Springs in Eastern Ruby Valley to cure various ailments. On occasion, family groups camped near the springs to use its curative water. If necessary, they carried the spring water to distant camps for use. Hydrotherapy also had advocates among nineteenth-century Euro-Americans. Genoa, the earliest settlement in Nevada, had Genoa Hot Springs where water cured 'rheumatic, cutaneous, and scrofulous affections.' The spring, a short distance south of Carson City, offered hot or cold mud and vapor baths supervised by a physician who helped the healing process.

Another form of hydrotherapy involved the use of the sweathouse by the medicine doctor. A small brush hut was made airtight with mud and the shaman placed the patient inside. Water thrown on hot rocks produced steam while a shaman with an assistant, sang and smoked a pipe. Sometimes, he buried the disease beneath hot rocks; at other times he buried it in ashes under a fire by thrusting his bare hands through the hot ashes, thereby producing a cure. Again, there are similarities in Western culture. North European cultures used the Finnish sauna or steam room for healing or cleansing of the body. The difference between Native American sweathouses and the Old World sauna is that the former stressed cleansing of the soul or spirit while the latter stressed cleansing.

PAIUTE

The territory of the Southern Paiute extended from a corner of California across southern Nevada, southern Utah and into northern Arizona. Many of the Southern Paiute's medical practices were the same as the other Great Basin tribes: disease–object intrusion, soul loss, sorcery, and power from dreams. To remove a disease-producing object, the shaman lay beneath the patient and removed the object by sucking. Both Southern Paiute and Northern Shoshone used chanting, drums and dancing by the medicine man in the healing ceremony. Various paraphernalia used by the medicine doctor was contained in his medicine pouch. Although most were crude or simple items– a cane, body paint, eagle claw, deer dewclaw, pipe, rattle or even a stone gave great power to the healer. and were indicative of supernatural power.

Tobacco when smoked by the Native American was used for ritualistic, medicinal and religious purposes. Limited to small amounts on infrequent occasions, it is doubtful that there were any harmful effects to the natives who inhaled the smoke through their noses. It remained for the new immigrants to abuse and spread the habit throughout the world. As a consequence the World Health Organization estimates that approximately 750 million individuals will have significant health problems from the use of cigarettes. This is true revenge for the introduction of the many infectious diseases by the new inhabitants to American natives.

WASHOE

The Washoe occupied the western slope of the Great Basin. Though they predated the other tribes in the region and belonged to a different language group, they shared many beliefs, including sorcery and object intrusion as a cause of disease. Sorcery caused most disease and could be produced by evil doctors.

A shaman had a special relationship with the spirit power (*wegeleyu*). The power manifested itself to an individual and it took three to five years under a senior shaman to become a shaman. Healing objects of the profession were: cocoon rattles made under the guidance of a dream; eagle feathers bound with buckskin; various items such as miniature baskets, stone mortars, bird-bone whistles, tobacco pouches, and stone pipes; also included were elaborate costumes used with red and white body paint, and headdresses, worn by the shaman.

For a healing ceremony the family paid in advance with buckskin, ornaments, or baskets. (The Washoe were the expert basket makers of the Great Basin). The ritual took four nights and was open to the public. With the patient's head to the west, the shaman blew smoke over the body. He then danced and sucked the object out or blew a whistle to invoke the cure. Sometimes he passed out and then coughed up the object, holding it out for all to see. The patient was washed and rubbed with sage. At the end of the cure, a feast was held. If the patient was not cured or died the pay was returned. They then hired another shaman to neutralize the sorcery of the first shaman. If too many patients died after treatment by an individual shaman they killed him.

SUMMARY:

Chemical analysis has found pharmacologically active ingredients and led to isolation and synthesis of related compounds. In a new industry, "chemical prospecting," current researchers are studying plants in the Great Basin. The herbal methods used by the Native American doctor worked for many diseases. Many cures sold to the American public by 'doctors' or purveyors of patent medicine in the nineteenth century had no efficacy. Native American medicine placed a strong emphasis on the psychology of healing, a potent ingredient in the healing process. With some exceptions such as surgery and vaccinations, the Native American doctor provided a service to his patient that compared favorably to medicine delivered to the average American during the frontier days of the West.

Vol. VII, Nos. 1, 2, & 3, 1996

WASHOE HERBAL REMEDY
For Mass Murder

David Prosser, UNRSOM Student

History of a Disease Winning Essay

The 1918 flu pandemic has gone down in history as one of the most devastating diseases to sweep the world. Although commonly known as the Spanish Flu due to its misperceived severity and beginning in Spain where it was uncensored and more widely publicized, the first documented cases actually occurred in the United States at Camp Funston, Kansas.

In two years roughly one third of the world's population and twenty-eight percent of Americans had contracted the virus. It is estimated that 675,000 Americans died due to contracting the virus, a number ten times greater than the number of Americans who died in World War I. Though these numbers paint the picture of a disease that left no stone unturned, a small Native American tribe in Northern Nevada may in fact have been the most successful population in combating the disease by employing a simple herbal remedy extracted from the root of *Lomatium dissectum*, a plant indigenous to the Great Basin.

As the state with the smallest population in 1918, Nevada was lacking the infrastructure manpower to reach the sparsely located rural populations comprising the majority of the population and was thus slow to report cases of disease. Once able to assess the spread of influenza, it was found that thousands of the state's residents had died from the virus. Though many of those thousands who died had been inhabitants of reservations, Dr. Ernst Krebs, a physician in Carson City discovered two striking facts concerning the local Washoe. The first was the fact that, though members of the tribe had become ill with the virus, not one member of the tribe died from influenza or its complications.

The second was the fact that the tribe had been using the root of the *Lomatium dissectum* plant to treat those who contracted the illness.

Lomatium dissectum, colloquially known as biscuitroot, is a rare species of plant in the parsley family that grows in semi-arid climates in the northwest region of the United States and parts of Canada. Up to the time of the flu outbreak, the plant had been used by the Washoe to treat all fever-causing ailments. The method used by the Washoe to extract the active product used for treatment was peeling the root of the plant, then boiling the root to skim the oil off the top. A large dose of broth containing this extract was then given to the patient. One pound of the root was used to produce the medicinal product and it was given over a three-day period to tribal members who had contracted the Spanish Flu. Within one week's of treatment, all patients reportedly had a full recovery.

Dr. Krebs conceded to the fact that the use of the plant and the survival of all Washoe tribesmen who were given it as treatment for influenza may have been coincidental. Further supporting the utility of this plant extract in treating influenza, however, was Krebs's report. It was found that treatment of these patients using the extract alone led to a full recover. Other physicians began using preparations of *Lomatium dissectum* to treat Caucasians who had contracted the Spanish Flu and found great success. Dr. Krebs even went so far as to describe it as the most effective treatment of that time in treating influenza and any accompanying pneumonia. He praised the plant extract for its versatility, recording that it was more efficacious at treating a cough and longer lasting than the opiate expectorants of the day.

He also noted that it was a bronchial, intestinal, and urinary antiseptic, and it also was able to slow the heart rate and lower the blood pressure supporting his assertion the treatment had great versatility, in addition to treating the flu, native tribes used biscuitroot for ailments such as the common cold, arthritis, tuberculosis, and rheumatism.

The constituents of *Lomatium dissectum* have since been determined. The plant contains furanocoumarins and pyranocoumarins, both of which have been shown to have significant antimicrobial activity. The furanocoumarins, for example, have been shown to be effective in inactivation of both dna and rna viruses, and they also have antibacterial and antifungal activity. Also present are saponins, which are present in herbs used historically for medicinal purposes. For example these herbs have been used as tranquilizers, expectorants, and antitussive agents. Ascorbic acid is also found in the plant and is thought to have immune stimulating activity. Coumarins, which have been shown to be vasodilating agents and thus capable of lowering blood pressure, are found to be present.

Lomatium dissectum has further been shown to have both bactericidal effects to varying degrees against some of the most common infectious organisms, including *Streptococcus pyogenes, Escherichia coli, Pseudomonas aeruginosa, Corynebacterium diptherium,* and *Mycobacterium tuberculosis.* When adjusted for concentration, these effects were on par with penicillin. In addition, another study testing the plant's bacteriostatic and bactericidal activity against 62 strains of bacteria and fungi found at least partial inhibition of growth.

As a result of the successful healing effects of *Lomatium dissectum* in treating influenza found both in the Washoe tribe and the subsequent trials performed by physicians, the plant enjoyed a short period of popularity with four manufacturing plants producing extracts. However, this period proved to be short lived, as its utility was somehow unable to catch the attention of medical professionals outside of its region of distribution. Interest in the extract waned soon after the end of the influenza pandemic and production on a commercial scale ceased.

The legend of the Spanish Flu and the devastating toll it took on the world is well known. Though modern day technology, in conjunction with the breadth of information concerning disease, allow, for the most effective methods of treatment to be employed, it can only be described as amazing that the seemingly simple remedy used by the Washoe tribe was so effective as to not lose a single tribal member to one of the most infamous viral infections the world has seen to date. A disease that took the lives of so many of the world's population was no match for *Lomatium dissectum*. In the perspective of modern day, whether or not *Lomatium dissectum* could have had a greater impact by reducing the death toll of the flu of 1918 throughout the American population under the right circumstances is a moot point considering the theoretical basis of the question. However, there is no denying the impact this one plant had on a little tribe in northern Nevada that defied the odds and cheated imminent death.

Vol. XXIII, No. 2, Summer 2012

EDITORS NOTE:

Dr. Ernest Krebs was born in 1877 and received his MD from the College of Physicians and Surgeons, San Francisco, in 1903. He was licensed in Nevada in 1904 and served in the Indian Service in Carson City.

CHAPTER IV:
CHINESE MEDICINE

Chinese merchants and laborers came to the Great Basin through the port of San Francisco in the mid-19th century. In 1860, there were only twenty-three Chinese in Nevada, compared to 7,000 to 8,500 Native Americans and 6,857 white immigrants. Twenty years later there were 5,416 Chinese, mostly males, in the state, accounting for 8.7 percent of the population. These new immigrants worked in the mines, construction projects, and built the Union Pacific Railroad across the desert and through the mountains. Afterwards, national and local movements of opposition forced a marked reduction of Chinese. Even though they supplied needed services necessary for western expansion, the Chinese suffered from discrimination and were forced to provide their own medical and hospital care.

Fortunately, traditional herbal doctors—China Doctors or Chinese physicians—also came to America and brought a well-organized body of medical knowledge based upon thousands of years of clinical trials, experiments, and careful observations. Unlike American folk herbalists, they were well schooled in their craft and had an organized pharmacopoeia. We will tell the story of Chinese doctors in Nevada.

CHINESE DOCTORS IN NEVADA

Anton P. Sohn MD

The professional Chinese physician in Nevada was a mid-level practitioner and the backbone of medical practice in the traditional social triangle.

At the top, above the mid-level practitioner, was the 'scholar-physician,' usually a member of the royal court, while at the lower end was the 'folk practitioner.'

Herbal medicine and the use of animal parts was the basis of treatment, but in addition to herbal medicine, treatment of disease has a long tradition of surgery. Chinese surgeon, Hua T'o, in second century ad and performed operations, including amputations.

Today the best-known Chinese practice is acupuncture, a practice that in the 19th-century was reserved for the royal court.

In the New World, Chinese physicians became prominent and influential in both the Chinese and American communities. There were several reasons for their prominence. In many mining districts there was a shortage of medical practitioners, and the Chinese physician fulfilled a need. In addition, for many illnesses Chinese medicine was superior to medicine practiced in the West. For example, it was more effective in dealing with female complaints, sexual disorders, and psychological symptoms.

Dating from the first century AD, the earliest pharmacopoeia of the professional physician, Pen-ts do clung, attributed to Shen-nung, contained 365 drugs classified either non-toxic and 'superior' or 'inferior' and toxic. The toxic drugs were reserved for serious illness. By the 16th century 8,160 prescriptions, made from 1,892 ingredients, were listed, and by the 20th-century there were approximately 2,000 described ingredients. On the American frontier, probably no more than 600 of these ingredients were available. Doc Ing Hay had a little over 500 herbs in the Kam Wah Chung Pharmacy in John Day, Oregon, a gold-mining town seventeen miles north of the Great Basin.

Although herbs, minerals, and animal parts were important to traditional Chinese medicine, pulse diagnosis based on careful observation was the basis for diagnosis and treatment for 19th-century patients. Using this method, diagnosis is made by taking the pulse at three sites on each radial artery. Each corresponds to a body organ and is further divided into a deep and superficial pulse.

Thus, there is a superficial and light pulse, known as *Fu*, and a deep and bounding pulse, known as *Chien*. The third and fourth principal pulses are *Ch'ih*, a slow pulse at the rate of 3 beats per respiration, and *Shu*, a fast beat at 6 per respiration. It was said that by the use of pulsology a Chinese practitioner could describe the symptoms without even seeing the patient.

The number of Chinese practitioners in the Great Basin or in Nevada is difficult to evaluate. Many did register their diploma with the county recorder as required by law, but many did not. Some even had their names printed in business directories. When the long arm of the law tried to prosecute them for failure to register, many juries were reluctant to convict the offender. In Battle Mountain, a jury refused to convict a Chinese Doctor who failed to register. It was obvious that Chinese doctors provided a service that was appreciated by white settlers. In a community in Southern Idaho most of the white women went to Chinese doctors with whom they had better rapport than with white doctors. Of interest is that years later, many of the checks that were given to the Chinese doctors were found to be uncashed.

Not all of the practices brought by the Chinese to the Great Basin were good. They brought opium smoking and opium dens to the fast-living mining and railroad communities. In John Day, Oregon, an opium den was located in Dr. Ing Hay's pharmacy. A Chinese laborer made $1 a day and spent 50¢ on opium. It has been calculated that fifteen-thirty percent of the Chinese laborers in Nevada were addicted. Initially the habit became prevalent among gamblers and prostitutes, but it eventually spread to the general population. Virginia City in 1876 enacted a law against opium smoking. Unfortunately, this was not enough to curtail its use. Hypodermics and parenteral use of opiates spread during the 1870s. Opium was even an ingredient in some patent medicines. An overdose of opium by use of the 'Black Pill' was used by the Chinese to commit suicide. A severely injured laborer, without support of any family, saw himself as a liability to his friends.

Invalids were unable to return to China suicide was the only way out—often with the assistance of friends.

Many Chinese prescriptions were equal to or more effective than some of the 19th-century drugs used by allopathic physicians. The realm of western medicine could profit from closer scrutiny of some of the ancient healing practices.

Vol. VIII, No. 1, Spring 1997

19th-Century Nevada Chinese Doctors and Location

Ack Sue Tong	Eureka 1880
Ah Gung	Eureka 1880
Ah Hung	Virginia City 1870
Ah Jet	Tuscarora 1880
Ah Kee	Carson City 1870-'79
Ah Lee	Elko 1870
Ah Quang	Ormsby Co. 1870
Ah Sam	Humboldt Co. 1870
Ah Sid	Wadsworth 1880
Ah Tong	Carson City 1877
Ah Wah	Washoe Co. 1870
Ah Wang	White Pine Co. 1880
Che Chung Hing	Reno 1880
Chin Guy	Reno 1880
Chin Pooty	Virginia City 1878-9
Chow E	Spring Valley 1880
Coke Sung	Virginia City 1878-9
Gim Hin	Virginia City 1873-9
Hing Ho	Virginia City 1886
Hing t. Wah	washoe co. 1890
Hop Lock	Virginia City 1860s-70s
Hop Wing	Virginia City 1875
Hope See	Ormsby Co. 1870
Hy Yick Chew	Tybo 1877
Jem Kee	Gold Hill 1878
Jim Hei	Virginia City 1880
Kee Carfung	Carson "City 1880
Kee Chung	Candelaria 1900
Kee Lock	Carson City 1880

Leing Shee Cheng	Washoe Co. 1870
Long Yut	Elko 1876
Men Lee	Eureka 1880
Mong Ho	Carson City 1880
Nung Kee	Eureka 1880
On kee	Virginia City 1877
Ou	Carson City 1880
Qort (illeg) Ahi	Ormsby Co. 1870
Quong Shang	Virginia City 1878-'79
Quy Fong	Virginia City 1871
Song Wing	Virginia City 1870
Tanig On Gek	Washoe Co. 1870
Tong Lee	Washoe Co. 1870
Tong Sing Tung	Ormsby Co. 1870
U. Wing Shang	Virginia City 1878
Wai Tong	Carson City 1899-00
Wan Gee	White Pine Co. 1880
Wan Quong	Ormsby Co. 1870
Wing Song	Virginia City 1878-'81
Wo Hing	Virginia City 1886
Wong Quong	Reno 1877
Yel Sam	Carson City 1880
Yon Haong	Virginia City 1878
Yuch Uh	Tybo 1880
Yung Hung	Carson City 1880
Yung Lin	Eureka 1880

EDITORS' NOTE:

An allopathic physician, also called a regular physician, treats diseases by conventional means with drugs that counteract the patient's symptoms. For example, if the patient has a fever or a cough, the doctor will prescribe a drug to reduce the fever or inhibit the cough. This contrasts with a homeopathic physician, who gives a drug that would produce the same symptom but in a minute dose.

CHAPTER V:
HOSPITALS

The first building called a hospital was thought to be on the Island of Cos *ca.* 300 bc and was managed by the Asclepias, a group of healers of whom Hippocrates was a member. The hospital had one hundred and eighty rooms and patients could stay up to two years.

In the 2nd-century AD, the monastery became the place where the sick received care, and the Crusades established hospitals in the Mediterranean and in the Holy Land. Their goal was salvation of the soul while healing the body. As a result, the foundation for modern Catholic hospitals was established. Later, lay individuals replaced priests, and still later, nursing became a profession. When the plague hit *c.* 1600 ad, the pest (pestilence) house was established to care for the sick and the poor who were unable to flee from the cities to escape the dreaded disease. The 'great' pest house in Vienna had as many as 16,000 patients, and it was a place of death and squalor for housing the poor. (Read Dante's *Inferno* for a vivid description.)

Some doctors in 19th-century Nevada had a room or beds in their office or home, known as resident hospitals, to care for a few patients. The concept of a hospital for the poor came into existence and remained a part of the American landscape (known as the county hospital) well into the 20th-century. Many of these hospitals had a separate or attached pest house for contagious diseases.

In the 1860s, civilian hospitals appeared in Nevada, and in the 20th century, the hospital became the treatment center for all citizens with serious illnesses or injuries.

On the other hand, construction of a hospital was the first priority when the U.S. Army established a frontier military post. Troops at Ft. Churchill built the first known hospital in Nevada in 1860.

Floor plans of hospitals at Forts Churchill and McDermit demonstrate a central hall and windows to accommodate ventilation as prescribed by Florence Nightingale.

WASHOE MEDICAL CENTER
The Beginning

Anton P. Sohn MD

Washoe Medical Center traces its origin to a Board of Washoe County Commissioners meeting February 17, 1862, when they reviewed a document stating, "Smallpox is prevailing" in the neighboring settlement of Watson's Mill. Although Watson's Mill was fifteen miles from Washoe City, the county seat, the threat was real. To meet it they levied a property tax of 20¢ for each $100 income to be placed in a hospital fund.

Also in 1862, the Territory Legislature passed a similar measure to ensure that indigents received medical care. They levied a poll tax of $4 on every man under the age of fifty, and gave money to each county to establish a 'pest house' for contagious (pestilent) disease. Smallpox, measles, diphtheria, and rheumatic fever were a 19th-century threat and swept through many mining and ranching communities. As a result of the legislative action many of the county seats built a hospital with a pest house, and many had a poor farm near or adjacent to the hospital where able patients worked.

Unabated, the smallpox epidemic spread through Washoe Valley, and in fact, throughout the West. Then, in 1864, the Washoe County Commissioners took positive action: Ordered that a committee be appointed to purchase the printing office building, or some other building, or build a new building, as they may think best for the interest of the county, and the same shall be paid for in scrip drawn on the hospital fund. Said scrip to draw interest at the rate of three percent per month until paid, in addition to the 10 percent per annum legal rate.

The Printing Office Building in Washoe City was purchased, and Dr. A. Gideon Weed, the first county physician was put in charge of the 'hospital' facilities. He was paid a flat fee of $2.50 per person per day to furnish supplies, medicines, food, fuel, and attendants.

By 1869 Reno had a pest house, but the living conditions were less than satisfactory, and the district attorney investigated the facility for criminal negligence. Three years later the allegations were still unsettled, and Reno was now the county seat. An 1872 grand jury recommended that Reno change its way of caring for paupers and indigent sick. The following year The *Nevada State Journal* on March 31, 1873, criticized the pest house, calling it, "A hog-pen, and a poor one at that." It was time to eliminate the problem.

On October 4, 1875, the Washoe County Commission appropriated money for: A small tract of 40 acres on the south side of the river (where wmc now stands), and 1 mile east of Reno, and 25 inches of water were purchased from A.J. Hatch for $1,000, to be used for a poor farm. On April 17, 1876, a contract was let to William Thompson for the construction of a county hospital on the poor farm, to cost $5,253. The building was finished and is now used by the county, being in charge of a physician appointed by the Board.

It was not possible to determine the exact location of this original building, until sewer connections and foundations were unearthed when a doctor's parking lot was installed indicate that it was situated along the Kirman Avenue side of the property.

EDITORS' NOTE:

References: County Commissioners Records, researched by the County Planning Engineer in 1930, and Myron Angel, ed., *History of Nevada with Illustrations and Biographical Sketches of its Prominent Men and Pioneers.*

Vol. VIII, No. 3, Fall 1997

FIRST UNIVERSITY OF NEVADA HOSPITAL

Roderick D. Sage MD

Nestled like a house between two hotels on a Monopoly game board, the University of Nevada Hospital graced the campus for sixty years, from 1902 until 1961. In the beginning it and its larger neighbors, Lincoln Hall and the Gymnasium, were three of a modest handful of buildings situated on the windy and barren hillside campus just north of the fledgling city of Reno. In the dozen years since 1883 when the University moved from Elko to Reno, there was minimal organized healthcare for students.

For a few years a rudimentary first aid station was available in the basement of Lincoln Hall, but in general sick or injured students would visit one of the several Reno physicians, or hope for a doctor's 'house visit' to their dormitory or 'tough it out.' As the student body grew to nearly 400 in the late 1890s, the need for an adequate campus infirmary became obvious. In fact, the Board of Regents had discussed this issue for so many years that it seemed to be a permanent item on their agenda. In their 1900 Biennial Report the Regents listed the five most urgent needs of the University.

1. Funds for the endowment of scholarships
2. An astronomical observatory
3. A natural history building
4. A library
5. A small hospital

President J.E. Stubbs recommended to the Regents a hospital construction sum of $1,500, but the state legislature, reviewing the funding needs, realized that this was a rather skimpy figure and wound up appropriating $3,500, which was adequate in that day and age. The new hospital was placed at what was then the north edge of the campus overlooking Reno. In 1900, each of the eleven college buildings seemed to stand specter like on the bleak desert landscape—in great contrast to the handsome, modern campus of today.

Preceded by Lincoln Hall and the Gymnasium, which were both completed in 1896, the new hospital construction was finished in 1902. Of the three buildings only Lincoln Hall remains—still a men's dormitory, and a venerable landmark second only to Morrill Hall in age and length of service to the campus.

The new hospital upon completion, was a 60 by 40 foot rectangular structure, and is described by the University Register…One story in height and with six rooms. Entrance is from the south portico into a reception hall. There are four wards, two upon the west for young men and two upon the east for young women. There is a convenient kitchen where food for patients is prepared and students are cared for by a competent nurse, and may have any physician they prefer? The 1902 yearbook, *Artemisia*, further describes the hospital as: Cottage like, of pressed brick with exterior trim work painted ivory white, a large door and windows, a sheltered verandah, and an indoor sitting room with an open wood fireplace.

The wards for men and women could accommodate five to ten patients each. Although architectural drawings for the hospital are not available, one can view a photograph of its exterior and imagine the appearance of its inner structure. Initially, a single nurse conducted sick call, cared for the hospitalized students, and staffed the hospital. After about 1930, two nurses were available to serve the sick and maimed. Students were allowed to stay for up to two weeks as inpatients, after which, if they still needed care, were discharged to their homes or to a local hospital. Students with contagious diseases were not admitted, but they were sent directly home or to a town medical facility.

In the 1920s, a local doctor was the university physician. In its first year the hospital got off to a worthy start, caring for 44 inpatient students, while 78 were treated in the school years 1903-1905.

As the university grew so did the hospital. In 1918, a basement was added, and just prior to World War II it was again enlarged at a cost of $10,900 to include two new wards, a bathroom, a sterilizer room, a closet, and nurses quarters. About this time the hospital became known officially as 'The Infirmary.'

Dr. Clair Harper, a retired (now deceased) Reno orthopedic surgeon, was the University Physician for years before and after World War II. He describes it as a 'jaunty little place,' where the young students were well cared for and the nurses were relaxed but always vigilant. His office was an enclosed square in the northwest corner of the central reception room, while the nurses' office was in the northeast corner.

A visit to 'The Infirmary' was described by the veteran Reno surgeon, Dr. Edwin Cantlon, who as a pre-med student in the early 1930s lacerated his finger in a chemistry lab mishap. The infirmary nurse cleaned the bloody digit, wrapped it in a snug bandage and sent Ed downtown to see Dr. Dwight 'Dutch' Hood, who at that time was the university physician. Dr. Hood unwrapped the dressing, gravely examined the injury, and then, turned to his desk drawer from which he extracted a quart bottle of Old Crow whiskey. He poured a drink for Ed and himself, noting, "This should make you feel better." After the doctor and patient both ingested the medicinal libation, Dutch rewrapped Ed's finger and sent him on his way. In Nevada of the 1930s, Old Crow was an excellent remedy not only for snakebite, but also good for all sorts of other ailments.

This dear little hospital served the university very well, until the ground that it occupied became more valuable than the structure itself. In 1961, 'The Infirmary' and its companion the 'Old Gymnasium' next door were both flattened to make way for the new Getchell Library and an ever-expanding campus-building program.

Vol. X, No. 2, Summer 1999

EARLY HOSPITALS
IN WEST CENTRAL NEVADA

Over the years there have been a number of hospitals established in the Reno area. Hospitals are created for many reasons, most of which are humanitarian, but teaching, response to epidemics and profit are all motives. When Dr. Bill O'Brien died last year [1991] he left some notes about Reno area hospitals that had been given to him by the late Si Ross, Sr. Mr. Silas E. Ross, a founder of the Ross-Burke Mortuary (now known as Ross, Burke, and Knobel Mortuaries) had an abiding interest in the history of medicine in Nevada. While doing research for a volume listing all of the physicians that had practiced in this state, which was published in 1957, Ross came across the names of many early hospitals. He gave the notes to Dr. O'Brien with the hope that they would someday be of value to medical historians.

The following is a listing of those hospitals, together with the information that Mr. Ross uncovered. We have excluded existing hospitals, such as Saint Mary's Hospital, Washoe Medical Center, Veteran's Hospital, and the more recent Sparks Family Hospital, because the history of these institutions is well documented. The remainder, however, are less well known, and we earnestly solicit any facts, information or pictures that our readers might have concerning these or any other Reno area hospitals. Please let us know if you have any such knowledge, and we would be happy to credit you with your contribution to this effort. Here are Si Ross' notes:

Adventist Hospital: Established 1907 at 804 Ralston; Dr. [H] McCubbin, Proprietor; Supt. Nathan S. Overton; changed to El Reposos Sanitarium in 1912.

Allen Maternity Hospital: Estab. 1919 at 544 N. Virginia by Mrs. Allen.

Bond Memorial Hospital: Established 1946 at 829 N. Virginia; closed in 1952.

Florence Crittenden Home: Established 1913 at 937 Forrest St. (now 1000 Plumas); it became the Sam Platt residence.

Royal Hartung Hospital: Established at 71 Ralston; Old People's Home for the IOOF and Rebecca Lodge.

Hudson Hospital: Established 1942 at 43 California Avenue; closed in 1945.

Invalids Hospital: Established 1904 at 519 W. Sixth Street; Cordelia J. Wentworth, Supt.; became the Wentworth Hosp. at 322 Chestnut.

Manitou Sanitarium: 141 West Fifth Street; Supt. Mr. Anderson; closed and the property sold.

Mount Rose Hospital: Established 1914 at 429 Granite (Arlington); closed about 1923; Dr. George McKenzie, Prop.

Nevada Sanitarium: Established 1923 on South Arlington Avenue; Dr. E.C. Galsgie, proprietor; closed in 1924.

Nurses Hospital: Established 1908.

Peoples Hospital: Established 1909 at Virginia Street at Fourth (2nd floor); Dr. J. LaRue Robinson and Miss Cunningham, Supt.

Red Cross Hospital: Established 1908; Alice Hopkins, Supt.

Reno General Hospital: Established 1929 at 429 Eighth Street; closed in 1933.

Reno Hospital: Established 1915; Alice Craven, Supt.

Rigelhuth Maternity Hospital: Lake Street near Sixth; Mrs. Rigelhuth, Adm.ag

Roosevelt Hospital: Established 1907 at 550 Sierra Street; Frances O'Hara, Supt.; later known as Saint George Hospital.

Saint George Hospital: Established 1904 at 835 Mill Street; Mrs. Lissak, Supt.; merged with Roosevelt Hospital at 550 Mill Street; Frances O'Hara, Supt.

Saint Mary Louise Hospital: Established 1876 in Virginia City; The 1st hospital on the Comstock.

Wentworth Hospital: 322 Chestnut Street; Cornelia J. Wentworth, Supt.

Whitaker Hospital: Established 1904 at 507 West Seventh Street; Property owned by Drs. Fee and Rulefson; Mary Evans, Supt.

Verdi Emergency Hospital: Built for loggers.

Gerlach Emergency Hospital: Built for gypsum plant workers.

Gerlach Emergency RR Hospital: For construction of the RR.

Wadsworth Emergency Hospital: Built for the RR.

Vol. III, No. 3, Winter 1992-93

EDITORS NOTE:

- Hardy L. McCubbin was born in Kentucky in 1864 and graduated from the College of Physicians and Surgeons, San Francisco, in 1899. He practiced obstetrics. He died in Sacramento, California, February 26, 1953.

- Edward Galsgie was born in New York in 1883 and graduated from Eclectic Medical College, Los Angeles, in 1914. He was licensed in Nevada in 1915 and died in Reno January 26, 1924.

CLARK COUNTY HOSPITALS

Phyllis Cudek, Historian

HEWETSON HOSPITAL

The Union Pacific Railroad System in Las Vegas laid the foundations for contemporary hospital care in Clark County with a tent community built in 1904 for employees. The company employed Dr. Hal L. Hewetson to treat ill and injured employees of the railroad in a four-bed tent located in the railroad yard, and it is believed to be the first Clark County hospital. In 1905, they replaced the tent with a permanent frame structure. This original building used by Dr. Hewetson for railroad employees was still standing in the railroad yards as of 1948.

LAS VEGAS HOSPITAL

Dr. Roy W. Martin arrived in the area in 1905 and later opened a six-bed facility, the Las Vegas Hospital, on the upper floor of the Thomas Building located on First and Fremont Streets. Dr. Martin also served a railroad, the Las Vegas and Tonopah Line, but also foresaw a great future for Southern Nevada and became deeply involved in its development. Dr. Martin's dream, however, was to build a new, modern hospital of which Las Vegas could be proud. With the assistance of Doctors [Raymond] Balcom and [Ferdinand] Ferguson, they acquired some land at the corner of Eight and Ogden Streets and broke ground for the first structure in Las Vegas designed specifically as a hospital. The building was completed in 1932 and soon thereafter, Dr. Martin and Dr. Ferguson turned to other ventures. Dr. R.D. Balearn, Dr. Clare Woodbury, Dr. Stanley L. Hardy and Dr. John R. McDaniel then acquired the hospital.

In 1942, the Las Vegas Hospital hired its first full-time administrator, Mr. L.W. Edwards, who continued in that capacity for over twenty years. After the war, Dr. Balcom retired, and three new partners joined the group. The medical staff consisted of Dr. Clare Watson Woodbury (surgery—urology), Dr. Stanley Hardy (obstetrics and gynecology), Dr. John McDaniel, cardiology and general practice, Dr. W.L. Allen (ophthalmology and otolaryngology), Dr. Grant Lund (pediatrics), and Dr. Gerald J. Sylvain (obstetrics and general practice). In 1959, Dr. Erven J. Nelson joined the group, which was known as the Las Vegas Hospital and Clinic.

The clinic, doctors' offices and the emergency and operating rooms were on the first floor. Fifty hospital beds occupied the second floor. The hospital had no facilities suitable for psychiatric patient care and did not admit patients with TB or contagious disease.

Hospital charges ranged from $7 to $10 per day for a private room; $5 per day for a ward bed; $750 for use of the delivery room; $5 to $15 for the operating room and $5 to $10 for anesthesia. Salaries for registered nurses in 1931, ranged from $75 to about $90 per month. The hospital closed in the mid 1970s. The Las Vegas Hospital Association was formed by various physicians to construct a "more accommodating hospital" at 200 North Eighth Street in 1930. This facility, the new Las Vegas Hospital, remained open until the late 1970s. Dr. Forest Ray Mildren opened his own Mildren Clinic in his home in 1930. Before the Boulder Dam project brought an influx of workers, Dr. Hewetson died and Dr. Martin retired. Dr. Clare Woodbury arrived in 1932, and with other physicians assumed leadership. Eventually the association dissolved, and the Las Vegas Hospital and Clinic emerged.

BOULDER CITY HOSPITAL

The Federal Government initiated the building of the Boulder City Hospital to care for employees of Boulder Dam and their families. "Six Companies," the conglomerate title given to the management sector of the six major construction companies working on the dam, built the hospital at a cost of $20,000. The Department of Interior requested that federal employees also utilize that facility. Medical and hospital care began on August 1931 under the direction of Dr. John R. McDaniel.

The hospital building was completed by Christmas. There were twenty beds including an orthopedic and a maternity ward. The cost of medical care for employees of "Six Companies" was $150 per month deducted from payroll, covering both employees and their dependents. This payroll deduction idea was the origin of today's Kaiser Permanente Plan, as Kaiser Corporation was one of the 6 companies building the dam.

Boulder City Hospital was located on a hill, while further down the hill a 'pest house' was built for isolation of infectious diseases. The pest house was a single large room filled with cots, surrounded by an 8-foot-high chain-link fence and treated smallpox, diphtheria, measles, scarlet fever, influenza and other conditions.

The entire complex was closed after completion of Boulder Dam. From 1938 to 1941 the hospital was converted into a National Park Service Museum and Office. It was vacated in 1941, but reopened in 1943 to care for wounded servicemen during World War II. The Bureau of Reclamation took control in 1948, and in 1954, deeded it to Boulder City. There was strong community support, with donation of money and volunteer labor to clean and rebuild used hospital equipment. Citizens organized a volunteer ambulance and the hospital continued to operate until a new hospital was built in 1974.

CLARK COUNTY HOSPITAL

In 1931, Clark County built the Clark County Indigent Hospital to accommodate the indigent patients from Las Vegas. For the first two years the indigent hospital was staffed by a single physician and one nurse, both on duty twenty-four hours a day, seven days a week. Dr. Hale Slavin became the county physician. He arranged for the construction of a surgical facility at the county hospital, and soon after that the hospital was renamed Clark County General Hospital. In April 1942, Dr. Jack C. Cherry moved from Goldfield, Nevada, to LV Vegas. He was immediately appointed house physician and administrator of the county hospital. As the only staff member, he was paid $150 per month.

Soon Dr. Joseph George was hired as a surgical assistant to Dr. Cherry. With establishment of a major military gunnery school in the area and the building of a magnesium production plant, the county transferred ownership of the hospital to the Federal Works Administration in 1943. After the war ended the county bought the hospital from the government. The population of Las Vegas increased rapidly after the war and there were a number of improvements in the hospital during the 1940s and 1950s. In 1956, the hospital was renamed the Southern Nevada Memorial Hospital to dispel negative connotations associated with a 'county' hospital.

In the 1960s, Dr. Harold Feikes, a thoracic surgeon, acquired a heart-lung machine that allowed him to perform the first open-heart surgery in Las Vegas. As of 1983, the hospital had a staff of over 300, and the only burn treatment unit in the state. Southern Nevada Memorial, later named University Medical Center, has developed into a major medical center in the western United States. It is now affiliated with unLVsom.

NELLIS AIR FORCE HOSPITAL

The U.S. Army Air Corps established a gunnery range at the site of the old airport in Las Vegas in 1940. Temporary barracks were erected to care for enlisted personnel training there. This was later relocated and developed into Nellis Air Force Base. In 1963, a permanent structure, the Nellis Air Force Base Hospital was built to provide medical care for military personnel and their families.

SAINT ROSE DE LIMA HOSPITAL

The Saint Rose de Lima Hospital was built in Henderson, Nevada, because of mining activity. A nearby titanium ore deposit, and the availability of water and power from the Boulder Dam lead to the establishment of Basic Magnesium Incorporated (BMI) in 1942. The Federal government required BMI to build a hospital for its workers, but by 1949 the defense contracts dried up, leaving Henderson with no support for the hospital. A Catholic priest, Father Moran, arranged for purchase of the facility from the government for $1.

The Sisters of Saint Dominic, a religious order from Michigan known for their success in hospital management, took charge of the Basic Magnesium Hospital, renaming it Saint Rose de Lima Hospital. The hospital served medical needs of the expanding community. From 1972 to 1981 it served as the VA Out-patient Center.

SUNRISE HOSPITAL

In 1956, Sunrise Hospital was started as a luxury medical center. Financed by the First Western Savings and Loan, and the Teamsters Union Pension Fun, it opened in 1958, catering to entertainers, gamblers, and wealthy hotel employees. Because the Teamsters continued to fund expansions of the hospital, it was often known as the "Teamsters Hospital." Sunrise developed Nevada's first intensive care unit. By 1966 it was one of the largest proprietary hospitals west of the Mississippi River. American Medicorp bought Sunrise in 1969. The management began an advertising program that included charge cards, 5.25 percent rebates for Friday and Saturday admissions, and recuperation cruises for Friday and Saturday admissions. The medical community had many ethical questions about the advertising campaign. Humana Corporation bought Sunrise in the early 1980s, renaming it Humana Hospital Sunrise. A Women's Pavilion/Neonatal Care Unit added in 1984.

COMMUNITY HOSPITAL OF NORTH LAS VEGAS

In 1960, Dr. Evert C. Freir started the Community Hospital of North Las Vegas to supplement Air Force health services. The hospital provided basic care for military families and hotel workers. After several expansions Huntington Health Services, Inc.

bought the center. A new full-service hospital was built in 1971. In 1975, the hospital opened a much-needed alcoholic rehabilitation unit. American Healthcare Management acquired the hospital in the 1980s and added a nuclear medicine facility.

WOMEN'S HOSPITAL

Dr. Quincy Fortier and Dr. Robert Porter O'Donnel provided a 'birthing center' with the opening of Women's Hospital in 1960.

Because of the high cost of new technology and treatment methods, they sold the hospital to Ramada Inn Corp. in the 1970s, and they in turn sold the hospital to Peresellsis Corp. in 1980.

DESERT SPRINGS HOSPITAL

Before 1970, the Desert Springs Hospital was an extended care facility operated by the Four Seasons Corp. The Charter Medical Corp. bought it and converted it into an acute care hospital. Dr. Hugh Follmer was the first Chief of Staff and Star Acuff was Director of Nursing. Because of its proximity to the Las Vegas Strip, the hospital provided care for many celebrities and entertainers as well as local patients.

VALLEY MEDICAL CENTER

In 1971, a group of local investors bought the Nevada Convalescent Center and renamed it Valley Hospital. After some renovations and expansion the name was changed to Valley Medical Center, and in 1979, it was sold to Universal Health Services. The hospital established an emergency medical helicopter service in 1980, and they opened an eye bank about that same time. The Las Vegas Hospital closed in 1974 and was destroyed by fire in 1988.

The economic and population growth of Clark County was affected by many diverse factors. The arrival of railroads and the construction of Boulder (Hoover) Dam, the establishment of Basic Magnesium and other mining developments, the Army Air Corps Gunnery range and later Nellis Air Force Base were some of these factors. The development of gaming and the resort hotel industry contributed greatly to growth. The warm climate, made tolerable by modern air conditioning, provided an atmosphere where people were encouraged to be the "new pioneers." The explosion of medical technology and the arrival of specialized physicians guaranteed good health care for the citizens of Southern Nevada.

Vol. IV, No. 3, Fall 1993

Vol. VII, No, 4, Winter 1996-7

EDITORS NOTE:

- Reference: "A History of Hospital: Clark County, Nevada," a master's thesis by Sandy Klimek for unlv, Department of Nursing, December 5, 1985.
- Dr. Wilmer Lars Allen was born in Utah in 1907. He graduated from University of Utah in 1929 and the University of Pennsylvania Medical College in 1932. He

practiced in Provo, Utah, before coming to Las Vegas in 1946. Dr. Allen was board certified in otolaryngology and served in the U.S. Army from 1942 to 1946. He was president of the ccms in 1951.

- Dr. Raymond B. Balcom graduated from the University of Nebraska School of Medicine and came to Nevada in 1930. He served on the bme and retired to Ontario, California.

- Dr. Stanley Laird Hardy was born in Utah in 1906, graduated from University of Utah in 1930, and Rush Medical College in 1933. Dr. Hardy was licensed in Nevada in 1933 and practiced in Overton, Nevada, in 1935. In Las Vegas he was a member of the bme, president of ccms, and president of nsma in 1957. Hardy died March 14, 1976.

- Dr. Grant Lund was born in 1905 and graduated from the University of Maryland Medical School in 1936. He was licensed in Nevada and registered in Las Vegas in 1946.

- Dr. John Riley McDaniel, Jr., was born in Mississippi in 1900. He attended the University of Mississippi and graduated from the New York University of Medicine Medical School in 1924. After practicing in Blytheville, Arkansas, he came to Las Vegas in 1931. He served in the U.S. Army from 1942 to 1945. He was president of nsma in 1946.

- Dr. Clare Watson Woodbury was born in Utah in 1895, graduated from George Washington University in Washington, DC, in 1923, and licensed in Nevada in 1923.

- Dr. Gerald Sylvain was born in Montana in 1909 and graduated from Marquette School of Medicine in 1933. He moved to Goldfield, Nevada, in 1934, and became the state epidemiologist in 1940. Dr. Sylvain was in the U.S. Navy during WWII. After the war he settled in private practice in Las Vegas and was president of nsma in 1955.

FIRST COMSTOCK HOSPITAL
SAINT MARY LOUISE

Cynthia Pinto, UNR Graduate Student

Saint Mary Louise Hospital was located in the Comstock Historic District in Virginia City, Nevada. This private hospital, including equipment, was completed in 1876 at a cost of $45,000 and was in the final stages of construction when the 'Great Fire of 1875' broke out, destroying much of the city.

Father Patrick Manogue, who received substantial backing from a well-known Comstock family, instigated construction of the hospital. The property for the hospital was purchased around 1874 by Mrs. Marie Louise Hungerford Mackay, the wife of

Comstock Baron John W. Mackay. Building the institution was a personal endeavor of Mrs. Mackay, and the project was encouraged by her husband, who provided much of the financial support for the construction and operation of the facility.

The hospital grounds, previously known as Van Bokkelen's Gardens, was a prime piece of land facing Union Street. The location of the hospital away from the town, in the eastern suburbs, was a significant factor as it afforded the patients relief from the dust and noise of the mines and mills. This distance proved fortuitous during the fire of 1875 as the hospital was one the few buildings to escape destruction.

Saint Mary Louise Hospital, operated by the Catholic order of the Daughters of Charity, was the pride of the Comstock. The hospital opened its doors on March 15, 1876, and Dr. John Grant was listed as resident physician, although patients had the option of retaining their own doctors. Sister Ann Sebastian Warns and a staff of five Sisters, as well as additional maids, cooks and housekeepers, provided patients with the finest medical care available at that time.

The hospital was supported financially by the Miner's Union. Each miner paid the sum of $1 per month to the union hospital fund. This served essentially as health insurance, providing the miners with prepaid hospitalization and medical care. John Mackay secretly matched this sum for several years, threatening to withdraw support if the Sisters ever revealed this source of additional revenue. Between 1876 and 1897 more than 1,500 patients were treated at the hospital. Patient records contain a variety of diagnoses ranging from nervous debility and drunkenness to cholera. Many miners were admitted for hot water burns and scalding, an ever-present danger for underground miners on the Comstock. By 1897, Virginia City retained only a fraction of its boomtown population. A staff of only three Sisters who found it necessary to beg for food, clothing, bedding and fuel in order to keep the hospital open now operated the once opulent facility.

The impending outbreak of the Spanish-American War made it apparent to the Sisters that they would have to abandon the hospital, as their services were required elsewhere. In August 1897 the Sisters were called home to Emmetsburg, Maryland, and the last entry in the patient ledger reads, "The Sisters of Charity left for good, Sept. 7, 1897." So marked the end of the first private medical care facility on the Comstock.

Vol. I, No. 4, Winter 1990-91

STEPTOE VALLEY HOSPITAL

Letter: March 8, 2011, Betty Bianchi RN, Ely

I came to work for the Steptoe Valley Hospital in September 1955 as a registered nurse. The hospital was owned and staffed by Kennecott Copper Corporation (kcc). I am not certain when it was built or opened but I believe early on in the kcc operation. There was also another hospital in Kimberly for another mining operation and I believe they may have been in operation at the same time. Steptoe Valley Hospital had thirty-two beds. There were four six-bed wards, one for male medicine, one for male surgery, one for female patients (medicine and post-operative care), and one for post-partum care. We had an additional four rooms, which were used as private or semi-private. These were utilized for labor, pediatrics, or isolation as needed. One delivery room, and one operating room were located on the east side of the hospital, which also included four doctors' offices, an emergency room, laboratory, X-ray facility, central supply, administrators' office, business offices, and a large waiting room.

Four doctors, fourteen registered nurses, an anesthetist, a lab tech staffed it, and an x-ray tech staffed the hospital. Three of the nurses were required to be operating room nurses. These nurses also staffed the er at night as well as OB and the OR. The chief of staff was the chief of surgery, and the other surgeons were his assistants. The kcc staff also included two doctors and one rn at both McGill and Ely. There was housing for each of them. One doctor came to Ely in the mornings to cover for 'rounds' and surgery schedule. There were a total of eight doctors and sixteen nurses.

We were staffed at night by one rn in the hospital and the or nurses were required to assist when necessary for any extra help. There was one doctor on shift and one on-call. The patients consisted of the employees and their families. Patients were seen in the clinic when available and next in-line. No appointments, no physician preference.

The patients paid very little attention to office hours. They came whenever [they wished].

The surgical procedures included gallbladder, hysterectomy, Cesarean sections, appendectomy, tonsils, hernias, and closed orthopedic procedures. Major problems were sent to Salt Lake City and transported by ground ambulance or most often by private car.

Housing was provided for all doctors and nurses. Food was provided for anyone, anytime. The 'on duty' staff ate together and worked together. This all came to an end when kcc closed down their medical responsibility and then provided the insurance program in 1960 or '61. They sold the hospital for $1.00 to the county. (Not sure on the price). Anyway the doctors went into private practice, and the county hired the nurses (a few were hired by the doctors), as were the lab & X-ray techs.

I don't remember the salaries, but it seems the docs were paid $600/month and the nurses around $250. But remember we had full room and board, but no overtime. We had a great time, enjoyed working together. The doctors were provided a home and the or nurses lived over the hospital clinic or in the house next door. The 5 houses still stand on the hospital property.

White Pine County opened the new hospital in 1969 with forty-three beds and named it the William Bee Ririe Hospital and Medical Center. Their website is currently not available, but you may contact them at #6 Steptoe Circle, Ely, Nevada, 89301. Dr. Ted Ross was the Chief Surgeon when I came. He moved to Gardnerville, Nevada, in 1958 or 1959.

LAS VEGAS TENT HOSPITAL
Dr. H.L. Hewetson

Dr. Halle L. Hewetson was born in Clarisville, Ohio, April 1, 1864. He graduated from the prestigious University of Pennsylvania, Department of Medicine in 1886. That year, he joined the U.S. Army. Later, he organized the chair of pathology and bacteriology in Omaha, Nebraska. This gave him the opportunity to become railroad physician for the Union Pacific Railroad, but because of poor health he moved to Kemmerer, Wyoming. In 1903, he became the physician for the Los Angeles and Salt Lake Railroad in Las Vegas.

From available information, he arrived as the railroad doctor in 1904 and was the first to pitch a tent on the site that is now Las Vegas. The tent was located in the middle of an alfalfa field in the vicinity of Fremont Street. At the time there were only two ranches, Kyle's and Stewart's, in the valley. When Clark's Las Vegas town site was opened with prices of twenty-five-feet lots going above the $1,000 mark, Hewetson attended the auction.

He established the first hospital in Las Vegas, which was located in a tent. This hospital later became the Las Vegas Hospital. Doctors Ferguson and Balcon became owners. During World War I, Dr. Hewetson was assigned to Fort Lewis, Washington, in the medical corps. At the end of the war he returned to Las Vegas and was county physician until his retirement. He died in 1930.

Vol. XVII, No. 2, Summer 2006

HOSPITAL FOR MENTAL DISEASE
The Beginning

Anton P. Sohn MD

The care for patients with mental disease in Nevada started off on the wrong foot. In early to mid-1860s "mentally deranged" patients were jailed. Even today the jail may be the first stop for such patients, but in 1867 the state decided to change and contracted with the California State Hospital in Stockton to care for the "indigent insane" for $10,000.

In 1875, Doctors Alson Dawson, Granville Huffaker, and Franklin White visited the facilities in Stockton and found the one hundred and fifty Nevada patients living in unsuitable conditions. Furthermore, Nevada was paying $5,000 a month to California to care for Nevada patients. The legislature in 1879 allotted land for a state prison and $5,000 for Dr. Dawson to investigate building a state hospital. After Dawson's initial findings and recommendations, $80,000 was appropriated to construct facilities to accommodate 200 patients, and Dawson became the first superintendent. On July 1, 1882, 128 patients were transported by train to the new hospital.

In 1883, when Dr. Simeon Bishop was the superintendent, the hospital had 140 patients, and 110 were men. Dr. Bishop's biennial report to the legislature listed a cost to the state of 79¢ a day per patient. Most of this amount covered housing and food, and very little went to psychiatric care. In fact, many patients entered the hospital because they had no means of support. Two thirds of the patients were European, and the men had a range of diagnoses including masturbation, heredity, typhoid, religion, fright, intemperance, jealousy, ardent spirits, weak mind, loss of money, solitary life, alcoholism, and disappointment.

Dr. Henry Bergstein became superintendent in 1895 and served three years. His reign is credited for stopping the custom of exhibiting the patients for public viewing and changing the name from Hospital for Indigent Insane to Nevada Hospital for Mental Diseases. Nevada's Hospital for Mental Disease moved into the 20th-century with dignity.

EDITORS' NOTE:

Reference: Biennial Report of the Commissioners and Superintendent, *Indigent Insane of Nevada* (Carson City, Nevada, 1883-1884).

CHAPTER VI:
DISEASE

The story of disease from the time of Nevada's founding until today is a book in itself. We will deal with the highlights, as told in the following essays. Suffice it to say that the proper diagnosis and treatment of disease has brought about the 'Golden Age of Medicine,' as demonstrated by the marked increase in life span during the period from 1850 (less the forty years) to 2014 (greater than seventy years). In 1850, disease was diagnosed by the patient's history and physical examination. Medical treatment was little more than a home remedy.

Most of the tools we use today to diagnose disease were unknown at that time. In fact, they are still evolving. Although a simple microscope was invented in the 1600s, the invention of the electric light bulb and the compound microscope in the late 1800s opened the door for examination of body fluids and tumors. Malaria was diagnosed as 'intermittent fever (cause unknown),' until the microscope in the late 1880s revealed the cause to be a blood microorganism. X-ray radiation, which made the internal examination of the body possible, was discovered in 1895 by Wilhelm Roentgen.

Smallpox and other infectious diseases were treated by little more than 'watchful waiting.' As we will see Persia Bowers' disease, even if correctly diagnosed, had no effective treatment. Rhonan's infected fractured bone resulted in Dr. Gunn predicting death. Hosea's foot infection was a death warrant. The widespread use of antibiotics to treat these and other diseases came about in the 1940s. Other measures that reduced the spread of microbes include the elimination of common drinking cups at sources of drinking water and the introduction of drinking straws.

Consumption, phthisis, or tuberculosis (TB) was the most common cause of death in the 1870s. Because of its slow progress, many doctors refused to believe it was due to an infectious or contagious agent. It was thought that families with TB suffered from an inadequate constitution. Furthermore, many cases were not diagnosed due to lack of postmortem examinations. TB of the skin was diagnosed as scrofula or lupus and the tuberculous granulomas in organs other than the lung were diagnosed as tumors. The disease was drastically reduced by the use of vaccination, pasteurization of milk, and the introduction of antibiotics to kill the organism.

Infant mortality was astronomical in the early 1900s. As you will see in Dr. Mary's oral history, the doctor was sometimes called too late to manage pregnancy complications, and abnormal presentation of the infant resulted in a disaster. In the early 1900s infant mortality was twenty per 1,000 deliveries compared to five per 1,000 in 2014.

To give further insight into life in the late 1800s, twenty out of 1,000 Americans died in 1870 compared to five out of 1,000 in 2014, which is greater than a four times decrease.

The 1918 influenza outbreak caused millions of deaths across the globe, and its presence was just as severe in Nevada. Treatment of the disease is still evolving with the discovery of anti-viral agents. We have immunizations against many viruses.

Polio, a life-threating disease of the 1950s was virtually eliminated by immunization. In 2000, polio was officially declared eliminated by the World Health Organization, Unfortunately, a few cases have been seen in Syria in 2014.

Illegal drug use, a significant cause of disease, raised its ugly head in 19th-century Virginia City as demonstrated by Schablitsky and Grimsbo's excavations. The problem of illegal drug remains overwhelming today and is difficult to treat.

1918 FLU PANDEMIC

Anton P. Sohn MD

The flu outbreak during World War I was probably the most explosive and devastating disease of the 20th-century. aids might be more disastrous, but it certainly didn't circle the world as fast or kill as many in as short a time. Interestingly, both diseases are caused by a virus and targeted young adults. Older individuals in 1916 had some immunity to the influenza virus.

Influenza swept the world in two waves during 1918. The first wave started in early March at Camp Fuston, Kansas. The second—more deadly—wave began late August in France and was spread by ocean shipping and returning servicemen. As a result of the second wave, many as twenty-five million and possibly as high as forty million people died. In the United States alone, at least 550,000 people died of flu and its complications, more than five times our military losses in the war.

Because of the sudden onset of symptoms and the virulence of the unknown organism, many experts suggested a bacteria or a combination of bacterial etiologies; at that time, little was known about viruses. Even if the cause of the highly contagious malady had been established, the treatment and preventive measures probably would not have changed, thus the outcome would have been the same.

What was the effect of the fall wave—known as the Spanish Flu because the disease was uncensored in Spain and therefore, more publicized—on Nevada citizens? We cite newspaper narrations of the flu in Fallon (*Eagle*), Las Vegas (*Age*). Reno (*Evening Gazette* and *Nevada State Journal*), Sparks (*Tribune*), Carson City (*Daily Appeal*) and the University of Nevada (*Sagebrush*).

In Fallon, 'about a dozen cases' were mentioned by October 5, 1918, and the 1st death, Hall Sumner, age thirty-seven, was recorded on October 19. By the end of the month, citizens were concerned about prohibition and the menace of alcohol, 'Saloons a menace to society, the industry of others, and aid to the Kaiser.' In December preventive measures such as facemasks became mandatory in the schools. Public gatherings were banned. The epidemic was waning.

Las Vegas was harder hit and panic soon ensued. Although the flu arrived in mid-September, by mid-October there were 140 cases with five new cases a day. The symptoms were headache, backache, fever, and bronchitis. Pneumonia was a dreaded complication. Doctors were overworked, hospitals were full, caskets were in short supply, and the local undertaker, C.B. Faust was in bed with the flu. By the end of November, new cases were ten per day and schools were closed. Flu masks of four to 6six layers of fine mesh gauze' were recommended to control the spread. By December 14 when the 'Dry' law was scheduled to become law (it was delayed by a court challenge) approximately fifty people had died in the LV.

Panic was also the order of the day at the University of Nevada in Reno. On October 15, 1918, even before there was an outbreak, a quarantine notice was posted. By the end of the month there were forty-five cases and 1 death, Private Wilbourn Stock. The second death was Coach Ray Whisman and the 'girls of Manzanita [Hall]' were making flu masks. By November 12, the situation had quieted down enough for the military companies–wearing flu masks–to march in a parade in downtown Reno, commemorating the end of the war.

Off campus in the Reno-Sparks area the first cases were reported on October 12 and a flag parade was called off. It was reported that eating 'plenty of raw onions and food seasoned with red peppers' was a good preventive. Because the odor of onions caused people to keep their distance, this was probably excellent advice! Within one week everything was closed except the saloons. October 14 was 'Sermonless Sunday' and ministers were advised to use 'unpreached sermons' on the next Sunday. Milder than onions, sagebrush tea—an old Indian remedy, which breaks fever in hours—was recommended to fight *la grippe*. At least 16 dead were reported in the *Sparks Tribune*. The *Carson City Daily Appeal* reported that calomel citrate of caffeine, along with well-lighted and ventilated rooms with wide-open windows might be effective.

Dr. W.H. Hood of the State Board of Health promised help from the state if needed.

One can see that confusion and panic was the order of the day during the epidemic. The flu pandemic of 1918 is remembered in this country as much as is the horror of World War I. We can readily understand the concern of Nevadans in 1918, if we consider deaths due to influenza. The cause of the disease was unknown. and it outnumbered combat fatalities.

EDITORS' NOTE:
See the essay, "Washoe Herbal Remedy for Mass Murder" in Chapter III.
Reference: Phillip I. Earl

Vol. II, No. 2, Summer 1991

NINETEENTH-CENTURY HOME REMEDIES

Anton P. Sohn MD

Many cultural groups rely on the use of home remedies rather than treatment by a doctor. Consultation with family or friends for advice on medical problems is a natural process. Since acquaintances might have had similar problems that yielded to practical and accessible remedies, their advice was usually sought and followed. In the Great Basin, travelers, ranchers, miners, and settlers followed this simple natural process.

In fact, today, we would consider much of what the educated civilian doctor practiced in the nineteenth century to be little more than application of home remedies. In Austin, Nevada, Dr. Riddle in 1868 treated typhoid fever with mustard baths and brandy rubs, an acknowledged Basque home remedy. It is reasonable to assume that if someone else in the family showed symptoms similar to those of typhoid fever, they were treated in the same manner without contacting Dr. Riddle. In a setting such as the Great Basin, professional medical care was frequently days away, in one of six populated areas.

Due to the sparse population in the 19th-century West, the philosophy of self-help was prevalent to a much greater extent than in modern times. Even today in remote areas of the Great Basin it is necessary to rely on home remedies.

When doctors were not available, the first white travelers in the Great Basin had to rely on their own medicine chest or get various drugs from other members of the party. A variety of medicines were available and were carried by the immigrants. One important group of drugs was narcotic—morphine, laudanum, opium, or Dover's powders—used for sedation, analgesia and to treat diarrhea. A second group included purging agents. To achieve this effect, calomel (mercurous chloride) was administered for a number of ailments. Similarly, cream of tartar with antimony, Epsom salts, and castor oil were used.

A third important group comprised the alcohol solutions, which were considered to be stimulants. Alcohol was an important ingredient of patent medicines. Brandy, whiskey, and other spirits were used internally and externally. Also carried with the wagon trains were camphor, flaxseed oil, ginger, horehound, ammonia, carbolic acid, hartshorn, quinine, sulfur, turpentine, and many other herbs and chemical compounds. If the concoctions were not palatable, molasses, honey, and sugar were used as sweeteners.

When Raymond Doetsch crossed the Great Basin in a wagon, he described the medicine chest as containing, "Elixirs, tonics, salves, balms, unctions, and ointments, together with physiking pills, laudanum, calomel [mercurous chloride], essence of peppermint, castor oil, and patent medicines."

Just as important as available medicine were the various health care guidebooks that promulgated the various treatments and philosophies of medicine in the 19th century. In

1769, William Buchan wrote and published the first self-help book, *Domestic Medicine*, in Edinburgh, Scotland.

Written to educate and inform the public on the prevention of disease, it appeared in America approximately one hundred years later, and became popular. Written for the 'rural elite' to treat their neighbors, the book contained description of the diseases and their symptoms, followed by their treatment.

Many other books were published in America, but probably the most important was John C. Gunn's *Domestic Medicine*, or *Poor Man's Friend*, first published in 1830. Gunn, an educated physician, thought that every aspect of medicine could be practiced by the common man if the practice of medicine was reduced, "to principles of common sense.' He directed his treatise, "for families of Western and Southern States."

Many sects and ethnic groups relied on remedies indigenous to their culture. Latter Day Saints (Mormons) settled in wide areas of the Great Basin before and during the mining explorations, while the Basques came later with the growing sheep industry. Both of these groups had home remedies passed down by their elders. A typical old world Basque remedy consisted of a mixture of dried mustard and wood ashes added to hot water for soaking feet to ward off a cold. Whiskey rubs were also utilized by applying them to the chest, as were kerosene and lard plasters. Sore throats were treated hot water with ashes and mustard.

A Basque remedy for earache involved plugging the ear with a cotton pledget after blowing smoke into the ear canal. Warm cooking oil was sometimes used in the ear instead of smoke. Garlic and vegetable oil were applied to boils, and the patient drank the purulent material extracted from the boil to affect a cure.

Garlic had wide use in Basque medicinal culture. Internally, it was used in soup to cure the common cold and externally, garlic cloves were bound to wounds to promote healing. Poultices were also made of bread dough, wrapped in a towel or sock, and applied to the sore neck or afflicted area.

Many Basques used superstition and magic to cure conditions such as warts.

To affect a cure, a potato was cut into four pieces to simulate a cross, rubbed on the wart and buried in a manner reminiscent of Native American practices. Cow manure was used on burns, as were some local plants. Urine had wide usage in Mormon folklore. It was used to treat chapped skin, sore eyes, earache, and was given internally to babies with the croup. Baby urine was also applied to normal skin to improve complexion.

In addition to the use of excreta, pioneer Mormon home remedies included the use of animals and animal parts. Brains were rubbed on the gums of a child perceived to be suffering from teething. Chicken liver was rubbed on a wart, and the liver was then buried in a manner similar to Basque treatment. Live animals were also used to treat serious and life threatening illness. Live chickens or pigeons were split open and applied to the chest as a poultice to treat pneumonia or applied to treat diphtheria.

More important to Mormon tradition was the use of herbs, sagebrush, and the divinely inspired 'Brigham Tea.' Widely used throughout the Great Basin, Brigham Tea was made from several plants, but the most important ingredient was a septated-reed-like grass known as ephedra viderens that contains a mild stimulant, ephedrine. Teas made from this plant and the common sagebrush was not only ingested, but they were also used topically on sores, sprains and in poultices. They were used as stimulants and tonics in the spring to purify the blood. Women used sagebrush tea to wash, invigorate and rejuvenate their hair.

Vol. VIII, No, 2, Summer 1997

1952 POLIO EPIDEMIC

Anton P. Sohn MD

Previous to the development of the polio vaccine by Jonas E. Salk in 1955, poliomyelitis was a dreaded disease of children, who were usually stricken between four and fifteen years of age. There was a greater incidence of polio infection following tonsillectomy, and this operation was frowned upon during the summer season.

Public gatherings were discouraged and organized summer sports were virtually banned. The poliovirus was endemic worldwide and occurred in epidemic proportions in the United States during the summer months. Reno was no exception and as the result of two near fatalities from bulbar spinal poliomyelitis in 1952 and 1953, a team was formed by wcms to manage future cases, since there were no available facilities between Los Angeles and Salt Lake City. The team included representatives from many disciplines. Maida Pringle represented nursing together with nurses Alma 'Red' Johnson and Reva Cunningham. One nurse, Renee Quinn, herself a recovered victim of bulbar polio, returned to work on the hospital team. All of the nurses did yeomen's duty, and in a sense pioneered in the development of the first real intensive care unit. Mr. Clyde Foxx was the wmc hospital administrator, and Ed Sontag was the hospital engineer. Actually, the first two patients treated with iron lungs were in the administrator's office.

Doctors Ken Maclean, Fred Anderson, Bill Tappan, Frank Russell, Wesley W. Hall. (Wes was president of the AMA in 1971), Ed Cantlon, and Vernon Cantlon were all general surgeons on the team, and Doctors Bob Locke, Peter Rowe, and Fred Elliott were the representatives from internal medicine. Pediatricians on the team included Jack Palmer, John Scott, Sr., and Emanuel Berger. The ent staff consisted of Joe Elia, and there were teams from neurosurgery, orthopedics, and anesthesiology. As a practical matter, the entire staff of wmc participated in the effort, and responded whenever asked to help. Dr. William O'Brien III, an anesthesiologist, spearheaded the project. The Washoe County program, which became a nationwide model, included training, fundraising, transport, ventilation, respiratory assistance–tracheostomy when necessary—and supportive care. Dr. O'Brien and his associates, Arthur E. Scott, Robert C. Crosby, and William E. Simpson described the program in *Diagnosis and Treatment of the Acute Phase of Poliomyelitis and its Complications*, published by The Williams and Wilkins Company.

As the first order of business, wcms established a 'Polio Equipment Fund' and a panel of its members appeared before service clubs in the area requesting support. Funds were badly needed to purchase iron lung type respirators, which at that time were the only thing available to care for patients with respiratory paralysis. Multiple sets of tracheostomy tubes and similar special equipment were needed to deal with the numerous cases seen in an epidemic. Civic leaders were taken to the wards of wmc to be shown the status of care and the need for equipment. The needed funds were quickly raised.

One person who was particularly successful during the fund raising drive was Barbara Savoy, who at that time was the office manager for the partnership of O'Brien, Scott, Crosby, and Simpson. Barbara was able to scrounge equipment from all over the United States. She was active in both the local and state March of Dimes organizations, and was able to arrange financial assistance from that organization as well. Washoe Medical Center was designated as a regional polio treatment center, and accepted patients from as far away as Grass Valley, California, and Las Vegas, Nevada. At one time the hospital cared for a maximum of eighteen patients on respirators, along with a number of other polio victims who did not require assistance breathing.

Some of the funds were used to equip the transport team, which consisted of an otorhinolaryngologist, anesthesiologist and hospital engineer. Forty-one patients were transported from 33 to 300 miles by air, ambulance or car. The ages ranged from seven weeks to fifty-nine years and there were few complications associated with the transport. A brother and sister about five and seven years of age from Grass Valley, both about one week post-op after a tonsillectomy and adenoidectomy, were stricken with polio. Since no care was available in the entire Sacramento area, they had to be transported to Reno, which was no easy task since U.S. #40 over Donner Summit was virtually closed by a blizzard.

The boy expired during the trip. The desperately ill girl, although she required tracheostomy and respirator care for a long time, eventually did make a good recovery. For the most part, many lives were saved by earlier respiratory assistance.

The success of the team is demonstrated by the statistics from the first two years. During that time 137 patients with polio were admitted to Washoe Medical Center and forty required a respirator. During the first year, the mortality rate for those patients on the respirator was 30 percent while the second year the mortality rate dropped to 17.3 percent.

The success of the polio team, in response to this medical emergency was due in part to the efforts of the community and medical profession. The various agencies worked together to identify, finance and fight what had been a nearly hopeless medical entity - respiratory paralysis due to polio.

Vol. III, No. 2, Fall 1992

Letter from Dr. W.E. Simpson Jr., Anesthesiologist

One of our problems was that tracheostomy. The surgeons had all been taught to do low tracheostomies so as to keep the tube as far away as possible from the vocal cords. However, a high tracheostomy made respirator care much easier, for suctioning, cleaning etc. We, the anesthesiologists, preached for a high trach. The word got around, since one day we got a patient. I believe a serviceman, from the Las Vegas area who arrived with a tracheostomy in place. He made a good recovery but was still unable to talk. After quite a while, Bill O'Brien did a direct laryngoscopy and found that, indeed, the tracheostomy was high. The tube was passing between the vocal cords.

We also had an infant who required tracheostomy and respirator use. After a couple of weeks the baby started having periodic episodes of respiratory distress. It finally dawned on all of the fancy specialists, anesthesiologists, pediatricians, surgeons, etc. that even though the baby had polio, it was still growing and had outgrown the tracheostomy tube. At least twice, it was necessary to replace the tube with a longer one. The press soon learned that we were caring for an infant, and we received a donation of a baby-sized iron lung. I believe it was from either Harold's Club or Harrah's. It may still be rattling around in the basement or attic of wmc.

I was on call when we admitted a husky, strapping, red haired young man who had been deer hunting in the early California season when it was still quite warm. He had shot a small buck and had carried it on his back several miles to his car. He was admitted with minimal symptoms of spinal polio in his legs. Over the next ten or twelve hours the disease rapidly overcame his entire nervous system. Tracheostomy and respirator care were to no avail, and he died around 4 or 5 A.M. I thought that this young man's worst luck was shooting that deer and the extra exertion from packing the animal out, for I thought that the exertion made his disease worse.

I recall a patient that Dr. Elmer Hanson flew from Hawthorne. Elmer had gotten a large plane from the Navy Air Station near Hawthorne. He had hand pumped the respirator all during the flight. We met the plane at the Reno airport and transported the patient to wmc, but despite all of our efforts, he died within a short time.

Vol. III, No. 2, Fall 1992

1922 DIABETES
PROFESSOR NATHANIAL WILSON IV

Barbara Parish, UNR Nursing Student

In 1922, Nathanial Wilson IV was diagnosed as a diabetic. At that time diabetes was almost always a fatal disease. Wilson was a chemist by profession and had moved in 1889 to become a professor of chemistry at the new land grant University in Reno, Nevada.

At the time, dietary management was the only known method of treating diabetes mellitus. His family relates how he would sit at the kitchen table with his scales, carefully measuring every gram of food that he consumed. At the onset of his illness he had been a short man of stocky build, but he soon became thin and gaunt.

He would test his urine for sugar by placing a specimen into a test tube, adding Benedict s reagent (a copper reduction test) and heating the test tube in a double boiler. The test tube would almost always turn from green to brown, an indication of high glucose. He would then attempt, by dietary management, to lower his glucose enough to enable him to function.

In 1927 or 1928, he was approached by Dr. Dinsmore, from the Nevada State Hygiene Laboratory and was asked if he was willing to be a guinea pig in an experiment. Two of Dr. Dinsmore's associates from Canada, Drs. Banting and Best, were attempting to develop insulin for human use. Wilson, by then, was tired of the strict dietary constraints immediately agreed to participate in the experiment, and became one of the first humans to receive insulin therapy. He remained insulin dependent until his death in 1961 at ninety-two.

Many of the local physicians referred their diabetic patients to Professor Wilson for help in managing their disease. He was aware of the difficulties that these patients would experience with wound healing, and was quick to provide them with Unguentum, a salve he had concocted and patented. He took great care with his own skin, especially the skin of his feet, and was quick to treat any injury that he might sustain with the same salve.

At the time of his death he suffered some loss of vision, but otherwise had none of the other usual complications of diabetes.

Professor Wilson, together with one of his colleagues, did work on the early development of X-ray. They tested the effects of the machine by holding their little fingers under the machine. Eventually, the repeated exposure to uncontrolled doses of x-ray caused great tissue destruction, with resulting atrophy so that the fifth fingers looked like 'a dried up claw.' Wilson refused to allow amputation of the digit, fearing that due to his diabetes the wound would not heal.

On one occasion the professor came staggering home with the assistance of a neighbor, who assumed that he was drunk. Although his daughter did not realize that he was suffering from insulin shock, all that she could think of to do for him was to give him a piece of chocolate cake and some apple sauce that she had just made. After this very effective treatment the professor rallied. He asked his daughter how she knew what to do, and all that she could tell him, "It just seemed to be the right thing to do."

EDITORS' NOTE:

- This interesting look at the early treatment of diabetes mellitus was taken from an essay written by student nurse Barbara Parish for one of her nursing classes. Her instructor, Susan Ervin, RN, encouraged her to submit her essay to *Greasewood Tablettes*.

- Ms. Parish informs us that Nathanial Wilson IV was her great grandfather. His son Nathanial Wilson V was a 1913 University of Nevada graduate who became a pharmacist, working in a pharmacy until well into his 80s.

- One of Nathanial V's sons, Frank (Tim) became a State Drug and Dairy Inspector in Nevada and his only surviving child is Ruth, the widow of the late James 'Rabbit' Bradshaw, a Hall of Fame football player at UNR.

- Professor Wilson led an active and productive life. He achieved some measure of fame when he and his wife took their three-year-old son (Nat V) on a twelve-day bicycle trip from Los Angeles to San Francisco in 1894 accompanied by a friend, Miss Bertha Bender.

- Banting and Best were co-discovers of insulin. Frederick Banting was awarded the Nobel Prize for Medicine in 1923. He was so incensed that his junior partner, Charles Best, was not recognized for his contribution to the research that he gave half of the prize money to Best.

Vol. IV, No. 1, Spring 1993

DEALING WITH SMALLPOX

Smallpox was just one of the devastating infectious diseases immigrants introduced into the West, and it was introduced into native Paiute and Washoe tribes. When it appeared the Department of the Interior provided funds for vaccination. In some situations, the Army was expected to provide the service free of charge, but when the disease outbreak was not near a military installation, the Department hired civilian physicians to do the vaccinating.

Dr. George Munckton was one of the earliest doctors to practice medicine in Carson City. Dr. Munckton practiced there from 1859 until 1878. He was also a volunteer surgeon at Fort Nye (near Carson City) in 1864. During the period from 1863 until 1865 he vaccinated 416 Indians to protect them from smallpox. The local Indian agent submitted a request for payment to Dr. Munckton in 1868—three years after Munckton's treatment.

The following letter to the commissioner accompanied a bill to pay Dr. Munckton $916, one dollar for each Indian and $500 for the service.

Hon. N.G. Taylor, Commissioner of Indian Affairs,

Wash. D.C. July 21, 1868

Sir,

I have the honor to submit herewith a subsequent account for the consideration of the Department. 1 designed to have this account accompany my final account submitted and settled during the post month. Unfortunately I did not have this account with me. I had ordered it sent here in time for it to make a part of the former account spoken of, but it did not reach me as soon as I expected it would, and desiring to settle my affairs so as to stop the suit that had been commenced against my Bondsman, I proceeded to settle the account then on hand.

The account against the Government arose in this way. The 'small pox' that was communicated to the Indians in their wearing cast off clothes, worn by persons afflicted with this disease. In this way the disease was very generally spread throughout the Pah Utah and Washoe tribes. The Commandant at Ft. Churchill was induced to employ his Sergeon [sic] to vaccinate the neighboring Pah Utahs, which he did, and afterwards presented a bill of some $2,000, which I refused to pay or in any way recognize. I told him that he was employed by the Government and that being in an Indian Country he should treat the Indians free of charge.

Dr. Moncton [sic] visited the different Indian comps and made an exceedingly low charge for his services. The necessity for incurring this expense will be understood better when I stay [sic] that the Indians were dying at a fearful rate, more than one hundred died at the Truckee Reservation. And in many other parts the disease was only arrested by vaccination.

Signed,

Jacob T. Lockhart, Late Indian Agent, Minden.

EDITORS' NOTE:

- Smallpox declared to be eradicated from the face of the earth in 1973.
- Bob Ellison of the Nevada Lawmen Research Project provided us with a copy of the original letter, which he found in the Records of the Bureau of Indian Affairs.

Vol. XII, No, 2, Fall 2001

NEW WORLD HANTAVIRUS

Chelsea Isom, UNSOM Medical Student

Disease with symptoms similar to the present-day Hantavirus has been described in China since 1000 ad. It manifested in frightening ways, with conjunctival hemorrhages, petechial rashes, edema, cutaneous flushing, renal failure, and death. Even with high mortality and unknown cause, the disease was thought to be self-limiting and not spread by human contact. In the 1950s this ancient disease probably reappeared in 3,200 American soldiers in Korea. Doctors described it as hemorrhagic fever with renal symptoms (hfrs). It would be over twenty-five years before its cause, Hantavirus, would become elucidated and found in the United States.

The virus was named after the Hantaan River in Korea, the site of the 1950s outbreak, but when much later, it occurred in the United States, it became the 'New World Hantavirus.' This disease presented with pulmonary symptoms and not renal symptoms, and hence the name, Hantavirus Pulmonary Syndrome (hps). By 2009, over 700 people were diagnosed in America. Nevada State Medical Association President Dr. Brian Callister documented Nevada's first case, and Dr. Stephen St. Jeor at the University of Nevada School of Medicine led the way with research. The following narrative tells the history of Hantavirus, reviews Callister's patients, and details St. Jeor's research.

In the 1950s, American soldiers stationed in Korea became ill with hemorrhagic renal syndrome with twenty percent mortality.

Doctors recognized that all of the soldiers had the same disease, but efforts to identify its cause were unsuccessful. In 1978, Hantavirus was isolated from a striped field mouse, and doctors concluded that Hantavirus had caused hfrs in the American soldiers. A survey of rodents in the United States determined that different rodents were hosts to different strains of Hantavirus. The common rat carries Seoul Hantavirus, and the meadow vole carries Prospect Hill Hantavirus. The survey suggested that Hantavirus in the U.S. had evolved within separate rodent species. After these revelations, researchers reviewed patients in the Centers for Disease Control and Prevention's (cdc) database and found 3 patients in Boston with a mild hemorrhagic disease, and several patients on dialysis with antibodies to hfrs.

On May 14, 1993, the New Mexico Department of Health reported three unexplained deaths among previously healthy individuals. Two were engaged to be married to one another and died within days of each other. Later, the Indian Health Services identified 5 patients who died from acute respiratory failure in Four Corners where New Mexico, Arizona, Utah, and Colorado meet. Investigating agencies could not find the cause, similar to the situation that had occurred in Korea. However, within eight weeks, ten people died from acute pulmonary failure in Four Corners.

All tests were negative, but cdc scientists using a test developed by the U.S. Army found antibodies to the Hantavirus. Researchers also found the virus in mouse excrement, and Hantavirus nucleic acid sequences were then detected in a deer mouse in the home of the first deceased couple. The new world virus was named Four Corners where it was discovered, but local residents rejected the notoriety. The virus was subsequently renamed Hantavirus Sin Nombre, which translates to 'Hantavirus Without Name.' Once the infectious agent was discovered, cdc researchers took steps to determine risk factors and focused on patients in Four Corners with unexplained respiratory distress or pulmonary interstitial infiltrates.

Less than three months after the 1993 cases in Four Coroners, Dr. Callister reported that two patients with Hantavirus in Nevada were treated by him, Chris Ward DO, and Hank Hayes, Physician Assistant. The first Nevada patient in July 1993 was a 24-year-old housewife from Round Mountain, who presented in Tonopah with acute respiratory distress. She had a one-week history of fever, myalgia, nausea, and malaise. When admitted she had bilateral interstitial infiltrates consistent with Adult Respiratory Distress Syndrome (ards). In addition, she had antibodies to Hantavirus. Up until then, clinicians treated Hantavirus with intravenous fluid and an antiviral agent, Ganciclovir, but they had 90 percent mortality. On the other hand, Callister felt that this disease was secondary to an overactive immune response, and treated his patient with high flow oxygen, aggressive diuresis, and high dose corticosteroids.

One month later a 51-year-old man from Tonopah developed fever, myalgia, nausea, and vomiting over six days. Within twelve hours after admission, he had rapidly progressing interstitial infiltrates, shortness of breath, and hypoxemia. He also had high levels of antibodies to Hantavirus. Once again, Dr. Callister treated the patient with oxygen, diuresis, and corticosteroids. Both patients fully recovered.

Dr. Callister related noteworthy facts about his patients:

- Both were treated at Nye Regional Medical Center in Tonopah, even though physicians in Arizona and New Mexico criticized Callister for not referring them. Yet, both patients survived while referred patients had 90 percent mortality.

- Both patients lived in absolutely filthy living conditions conductive to mice propagation.

- A guiding principle for Callister's treatment was his opinion that adults with intact immune systems develop acute respiratory distress syndrome (ards). For example, babies, elderly people, and immuno-compromised individuals rarely develop the syndrome suggesting that the life threatening complications of ards are indeed due to an over active immune response rather than viral toxemia. National guidelines now include corticosteroids as a treatment option.

After Dr. Callister's experience, by December 1994, there were 108 patients with hps, and over one half of the cases were from Four Corners. Most of these illnesses appeared in spring and early summer, which suggested environmental/seasonal factors. Researchers did not know whether this was a new disease or reemergence of an old disease.

In 1994, Dr. Stephen St. Jeor at the School of Medicine became interested in Sin Nombre Hantavirus. He learned about the virus from a friend, Dr. Stuart Nichole, who was in the special pathogen branch of the cdc. Dr. Nichole and colleagues discovered the virus in a deer mouse. St. Jeor and Nichole received a grant to determine virus transmission and investigate a possible vaccine. St. Jeor found the virus in 40 percent of deer mice in Nevada. He also found that workers at Truckee Meadows Community College in Reno had a terrarium of deer mice in their lunchroom.

Approximately twenty percent of the mice harbored Hantavirus; however, not one worker had the virus antibody. Even more interesting, the deer mice had been together for several months, but they did not have close to a one hundred percent infection rate as might be expected in animals living together in a cage.

In a closer-to-home tragedy, in the early 1990s, two faculty members in the College of Agriculture at unr contracted hps; one recovered but sadly the other died. When one looks at the difference in transmission statistics in the United States, the presence of Hantavirus in at-risk individuals (forest workers and mammologists) is very low compared to the carrier rate of the virus in deer mice. However, at-risk-individuals in Europe have a much higher infection rate than U.S workers adding to the mystery in differences in spread and immunity. Initially, evidence of the virus was found in salivary glands and kidneys, but it could not be grown in the laboratory.

Later, CDC scientists were able to isolate Hantavirus from deer mice but not from humans.

Dr. St. Jeor's study of the New World Hantavirus stretched from Reno's San Rafael Park to an Argentinean ski resort in Baraloche where the strain is known as the Andes Hantavirus. It is the only Hantavirus that is proven to pass from human to human. St. Jeor is trying to discover why the virus only occasionally affects humans and to determine how the virus is spread between rodents. In the U.S. the total number of reported cases is approximately 400, the number of cases in South America is over 1,000, and worldwide there are about 100,000 cases per year. Dr. St. Jeor is also working on the development of a vaccine, but because of the small number of human cases, pharmaceutical companies consider it to be financially impractical.

On another level researchers questioned why the 1993 Hantavirus had reemerged in greater numbers than in previous years. They desired to determine factors that would predict future outbreaks. It was discovered that rain enhanced food supply producing an increase in deer mice. In 1997 there was a significant early rainfall, suggesting to scientists the possibility of a Hantavirus outbreak. The department of health warned Four Corners authorities about the increased risk. Despite these warnings, the number of patients increased from six in 1995-97 to thirty-three in 1998.

The Sin Nombre strain of Hantavirus is present in the United States, and while it may not be widely reported in the news, it is still taking lives. In 2010, five children from Four Corners developed hps and one died. All five lived or played in areas near deer mice. The Sin Nombre virus is in Nevada, but if it will ever cause a large number of infections like the Old World hhrs strain is uncertain. One thing is clear, to prevent this disease one needs to avoid areas where rodent's droppings can be aerosolized.

EDITORS' NOTE:

- The hps virus-carrying deer mouse is brown, unlike the common gray colored house mouse found in homes throughout the world. On the other hand, there are other rodents that carry viruses associated with human infections, such as the Prospect Hill virus that is found in meadow voles throughout the world. The best advice is to join our wives, daughters, and granddaughters and avoid contact with all mice.

- Dr. Brian Callister completed his residency at ucla, and Nye Regional Medical Center recruited him with financial aid from the Rural Nevada Health Service Corps to locate to Tonopah. He knew Tonopah from refueling stops in the small airplane when he flew as a child with his surgeon father. During four years of practice in Tonopah, he cared for the patients with Hantavirus and also became friends with physicians from Reno. When he decided to move to Reno, it was because of his relationships and respect for those Reno physicians that he decided to relocate in Reno.

- Dr. Stephen St. Jeor, when a graduate student at the University of Utah, studied mechanisms by which arthropod-born encephalitis viruses, after being dormant, reappear in the spring. This research was instrumental in stimulating his interest in viruses found in nature. He worked with human herpes viruses for thirty years, both at the Pennsylvania State University's Hershey Medical Center and later at the University of Nevada School of Medicine, where he was working when the outbreak of Hantaviruses occurred in Four Corners renewed his interest in the spread of viruses. When his colleague, Stuart Nichol, who had worked at unr's College of Agriculture and the School of Medicine, moved to the cdc, St. Jeor remained friends. They later agreed to jointly study the new Hantavirus, which reignited Dr. St. Jeor's interest in the survival of viruses in nature.

Vol. XXII, No. 2, Summer 2011

MYSTERY OF LITTLE PERSIA BOWERS

Eileen Barker, UNSOM Pathology Office Manager

Nevada State Journal July 15, 1874, "Died—in Reno, July 14. Persia Bowers, 12-years old."

One hundred and eighteen years later the cause of this child's death remains as much a mystery as the circumstances surrounding her birth and adoption. No official records of her death can be found, and sources of information are few and mostly unreliable.

The story begins in 1859 when Lemuel Sanford 'Sandy' Bowers, a miner in Virginia City, Nevada met and married boardinghouse owner Alison 'Eilley' Cowan. The two held interest in adjacent mines. The mines struck silver and the money poured in. They amassed a fortune reported to be $4,000,000. In 1861 construction of a home suitable for the new millionaires was planned in Franktown, a lush valley lying between Carson City and Lake's Bridge (later renamed Reno).

At this point fact and legend merge. It has been written that the Bowers traveled to Europe, and for two years, cut a wide swath shopping and shipping home expensive furniture for the new home. The story continues that on the return trip aboard the *SS Persia* of the Cunard Line, while traveling from Liverpool to New York City, Eilley took as her own child the infant daughter of a woman, Margaret Wixson, who had died and was buried at sea. Eilley named the child Margaret Persia. Four years later, in 1868, following the untimely death of Sandy Bowers, the widow was engulfed in financial difficulties. Creditors and bill collectors descended on the heavily mortgaged mansion and chaos ensued. To remove her from the daily upheaval, Persia was sent to Reno, twenty miles to the north.

Reno was incorporated in 1869. Four years later, on Persia's arrival, the town was still in its infancy.

Persia found in Reno a flourishing clutter of saloons, stables, blacksmith shops, hay yards, stores, hotels, restaurants, several churches, a schoolhouse, a theater, a weekly newspaper, and a fire department. A handful of streets formed the town's business core with residential neighborhoods clustered nearby. Persia boarded on West Street at the home of N.J. Roff, a harness maker who also gave music lessons and played in the Reno Municipal Band. Persia studied music and prepared her school lessons. She was a good student at the four-year-old Reno school.

On December 20, 1873, the *Nevada State Journal* reported, "The usual closing examinations of the Reno Public School were held yesterday afternoon at the school house under the supervision of Mr. Orvis Ring, the very efficient teacher." The average attendance for this term has been about fifty. Miss Persia Bowers recited her composition, "Darwinism in the Kitchen."

As had been their plight in previous summers, during that hot summer of 1874, the citizens of Reno were plagued by fevers. Winds stirred clouds of dust from the primitive streets and rains turned the streets into quagmire. Most townspeople took untreated water from the Truckee River into which sewer lines emptied, or drew water from the irrigation ditches that lined most of the streets. The fevers—typhoid fever, military fever, swamp fever, typhus, cholera, diphtheria and malaria were treated with mercury compounds like calomel with doses of quinine, or with sweating the patient. Patients were also dosed with sulfur and molasses, herbal brews, lard or even axle grease. Despite the crude therapy some of the patients recovered, but many did not.

The doctor's office of that day was simple and plain. Prescriptions were compounded by hand. Surgery was performed in the patient's home, and asepsis was often ignored.

The *V&T Reno City Directory of 1874* listed four practicing physicians and surgeons—

Drs. William Bergman, Simeon Bishop, H.S. Brower, and C.W. Friedriechs. Dr. H.H. Hogan was the county physician with an office at the newly built county hospital and poorhouse, a facility for the indigent sick. The first general hospital on the Comstock was Saint Mary Louise Hospital, twenty miles away over Geiger Grade, which was a road to Virginia City. In 1874,it was still two years away from completion. Much earlier in 1861 Dr. Joseph Ellis had taken over a cluster of hot springs at Steamboat Springs, a few miles south of the Truckee River, and built a thirty-four-bed private hospital, which became a favorite place for miners from the Comstock to cure hangovers. It was not a general hospital in the usual sense, and in 1867 under suspicious circumstances it burned to the ground.

Hospitals generally were greeted with suspicion and fear by the people of that time, for being sent to a hospital was considered to be a death sentence. Reno citizens were no exception to this aversion, and they were slow to admit to the necessity for a hospital. It would not be until 1903-04 that a general hospital would be attempted, when an undertaker and veterinarian would renovate and remodel the old Whitaker School for Girls on Ralston Hill. This proved to be an unsuccessful venture.

In 1905, the Dominican Sisters remodeled their old school house, Mount Saint Mary's Academy at Sixth and Chestnut Streets into the hospital that continues today. However, for Persia Bowers on that hot July day in 1874 no such medical amenities were available. She developed a high fever, suffered intense pain and quickly died. Her mother, summoned from the mansion in Franktown, was unable to reach her daughter's bedside before she died.

What caused Persia's death? No certificate of death can be found, for the state of Nevada did not require the recording of births or deaths until thirteen years later. The popular belief is that little Persia died of scarlet fever, but certainly a multitude of other possibilities exist. With better medical treatment, could she have survived to relate the intriguing story of her family? It all shall probably remain a mystery.

Vol. 3, No. 1, Summer 1992

MEDICAL ARCHEOLOGY
IN VIRGINIA CITY

Julie M. Schablitsky and Raymond A. Grimsbo, Archeologists

Traditional methods of archaeology involve analysis of artifacts by date, description, composition, function, location, and analysis of the items. A difficult challenge for urban archaeologists is to assign ownership to artifacts recovered from household refuse where there is high-density population.

Julie M. Schablitsky from Portland State University and Raymond A. Grimsbo of Intermountain Forensic Laboratories, Inc., utilized dna analysis in the new subfield of forensic archaeology to study items recovered from an archaeological dig.

During excavation of a Virginia City working class neighborhood, they found the remains of a 19th-century dwelling. The house was situated in a densely occupied ethnically heterogeneous neighborhood in the 1870s. It was two blocks east of the red light district and adjacent to Chinatown. The neighborhood included European immigrants, Americans, and Africans.

The address, 18 North G Street, recorded in the Virginia City land deed book, appeared in 1873 as a dressmaker shop operated by Mrs. M.A. Andrews, a Daughter of the Temperance Society. In July 1873, Mrs. Andrews died at the age of thirty-five, and based on the lack of affordable housing in Virginia City, new tenants most likely moved into that address that summer.

By 1875, a British family, the Coopers, was living in that house. The crowded dwelling contained carpenter Thomas Cooper, his wife Eunice and three children. In October 1875, a large fire that razed central Virginia City destroyed the house.

Almost 125 years later, archaeologists excavating the charred remains of the house found many artifacts commonly associated with households such as bottle glass, buttons, beads, stoneware, and straight pins. However, there was an unexpected find. Discarded beneath the floorboards was a glass hypodermic syringe with a rolled copper needle. Six more hypodermic syringe needles were found.

The discovery of drug paraphernalia prompted the questions: Who used the syringe and for what purpose, and what was injected? The hypodermic injection of medicines, particularly morphine, became widely accepted across America during the 1860s and 1870s. Although other drugs such as quinine, caffeine, atropine, and strychnine were used, morphine was injected about ninety percent of the time.

Morphine and syringe kits were available in local pharmacies. Easy access to drugs gave rise to nonmedical drug use. Injection of morphine was more potent and less expensive than opium smoking. The effect of morphine on the body included a warm glow of benevolence, a disposition to do great things, and a mental calmness. The low cost and the sense of euphoria may have encouraged the social use of morphine. Dr. F.E. Oliver observed in 1872, "The sulphate of morphia seems to be growing in favor, its color and less bulk facilitating concealment, and being free from the more objectionable properties of opium." No social strata were untouched by morphine use and addiction.

Examination of four of the needles recovered during the excavation demonstrated human dna in two of them. The str (Short Tandem Repeat) technique suggests multiple users of the hypodermic syringe and associated needles. Additionally, male and female dna were found in at least half of the samples. Most intriguing is the presence of three loci most common in populations of African descent. These findings show that at least four different people used the syringe.

Schablitsky and Grimsbo suggest that a likely scenario was a social gathering of at least four adults where morphine was injected for euphoric effect. Recreational drugs were used on the Comstock. Forensic science has proved to be an invaluable tool to archaeologists. dna analysis and the str test in particular, have found historic data unattainable by the archaeologist and historian. The discovery of drug paraphernalia in the archaeological ruins of a house opened the door into the past, and forensic science has taken us through that door. What could never be found in history books is the physical profile of the drug user and the social setting in which the activity took place. The discovery of multiple users, presence of both males and females, and a probable link to people of African descent on the hypodermic syringe boldly illustrates the need to incorporate forensic science into the field of archaeology.

Vol. XIII, No. 2, Autumn 2002

SAD STORY OF THE GROSH BROTHERS

A drama with tragic consequence was being played out in Gold Canyon at Gold Hill. In mid-August 1857, the Grosh brothers, Hosea Ballou and Ethan Allen, were prospecting when Hosea accidentally struck his foot with his pick An infection ensued, and despite improvement after poultices of rosin, then bread and soda, a friend was consulted who recommended a poultice of cow dung. Dr. Benjamin L. King agreed that cow dung was the right therapy. The infection progressed and Ethan wrote his father, Rev. A.B. Grosh, requesting money to buy the services of Dr. Charles D. Daggett, the best doctor in the area. Unfortunately, the services of the "best doctor" never came, but Hosea's immortality was established. His treatment, although ill advised by today's standards, is one of the first recorded home remedies and one of the early medical treatments by a doctor in the territory that would become Nevada. The following is an abstract of that letter:

Gold Canon, Sept. 7, 1857

Dear Father,

I take up my pen with a heavy heart, for I have sad news to send you. God has seen fit in his perfect wisdom & goodness to call Hosea, the good, the gentle to join his Mother in another and a better world than this.

At the time of his death I had gone to see a physician in Eagle Valley, some fourteen or fifteen miles from here. It was very sudden—unexpected but very peaceful. Not a shudder, not a gasp, not a change of feature marked the parting of soul and body. He simply fell asleep. It was such a death as God blesses the good with.

The immediate cause of his death was the wound in the foot I mentioned in my last. It occurred about the middle of the forenoon of Wednesday, Aug. 19, by first letter-Today-the-20. He died Wednesday, Sept. 2. We were packing dirt from a small ravine to the right fork of the main Canon. I dug and Hosea drove the jack. We had brought no water with us for drinking and becoming thirsty (it was very hot.) I started down to the main ravine for a drink. I met Hosea as he was coming back for another load and told him what I was going for and that I had not quite a load dug for him. On my return he was setting on the ground beside the dirt holding his left foot in his hand. "I have done it now," he shouted as I came within hearing, and on my asking what he had done, he said that he had "struck the pick into his foot" "Why how in the world did you do it." I asked as I first saw the wound. It was a frightful gash. The dirt we were digging was only sixteen or eighteen inches deep, and, though it dug hard, there were but few stones in it. He smiled, and said that he hardly knew how he did it. He then pointed to a large quartz rock laying loose on top of the ground just on the edge of the hole. "Somehow" he said, "I hit that." He would not let me carry him to the house but rode the jack. The ground was rough, and the jolting caused him considerable pain. For about a week it got on finely, in spite of the hot weather. But the evening of the eighth day, his foot was swolen [sic], and the wound closed.

The next morning I lanced the foot in two places and got out considerable matter, which relieved the pain, and checked the swelling. I also changed the poultice from rosin soap to bread and soda. The bread and soda worked very well, and I think that if we had continued it everything would have come out right. Monday afternoon I went down to the store—four or five miles—to see if I could get either opium or laudanum, so that he might get his necessary rest. I could find neither, but I saw Mr. Rose, and he told me that he had some at his house in Eagle Valley. He also recommended me to try fresh cow dung as a poultice. I took some cow-dung up with me, and applied it immediately. I should have mentioned that the leg had commenced swelling, and that we could not check it. The poultice at once checked the swelling, and ...ed the pain, and next morning everything was looking well again.

I found a man who was going up to Eagle Valley and sent by him for the opium, and also for a little quinine, cayenne & several other things if they could be got. I could get nothing here & Hosea was quite billious [sic] besides touched with the dyspepsia—the result of his confinement to bed. I understood the man would be back that evening, but that evening found that I was mistaken. This evening also occurred the misshap [sic], which I think sent Hosea out of this world. The cat jumped on the bed, and in doing so lit with all his weight on poor Hosea's sore foot. It caused him intense pain. That night he suffered great pain, and next morning he had a high nervous fever.

He complained that during the night he had been slightly flighty. He was very cool and calm, and before I went to see Dr. King (formerly of Dearfield N.Y.) Sr with whom we had some slight aquaintance [sic] we had considerable conversation, He [Hosea] said, that "through God's mercy we had passed through as great trials as this—and to that mercy we must trust—without God's mercy what would we be?

Dear Brother! he spoke as though the trial was as much on me as on him. He was so uncomplaining & made so little of his sufferings that it took close watching to see how sick he really was. After some little thought he consented to a proposition I made to send to you for $50 or $100, so that we could, on the strength of it secure the services of Dr. Daggert, the only good doctor in Carson Valley, should they be necessary. Little did either of us dream of the danger being so near at hand.

I dressed his foot. It was rather cold. He quieted my apprehentions [sic] by saying that it was the effect of the warm poultices. The poultice was warmer, a little, than blood heat. He felt it very sensible, and we both congratulated ourselves on the favorable symptom, as the poultice before that had been warmer and he had hardly felt it. He complained of being ... sick", just before I left, but felt no other pain.

About 9 A.M. I started for Eagle Valley to see Dr. King and get what medicine I could, leaving him in charge of Mr. Galphins, who came to the house a few minutes after I had left. I had not gone far before a feeling of uneasiness took hold of me. Twice I threw myself down behind a cedar bush, completely overcome with a great dread that it would terminate fatally. I prayed—oh with what agony I prayed that he be spared—that the loss of the limb might be the worst. Finally to get rid of this dreadful apprehension I struck across the mountains, which though it shortened the distance a few miles, was very rough, and I was almost barefooted.

Dr. King was very kind to me. He recommended the continunance [sic] of the cow dung poultice, as being the best to be had here. He did not regard the swelling of the foot & leg—neither the coldness—as anything serious. He spoke spoke [sic] as if a wound got along very slow in this country, but did not seem to think that the danger was increased thusly. Hosea complained of pain in the back, and one particular spot, near the shoulders on the left side, he said produced nausea if it touched the bed. The doctor regarded it only as the resift of the pain and loss of sleep together with slight billiousness [sic] He gave me four pills of Blue Mass—which I took for fear of hurting his feelings. But I gotten or fifteen grains of quinine.

Though I could get no physic but aloes or Ep. Salts, both of which we had and would not use. I regretted very much that I could get no hops, as I had more hope of allaying the nausea with that than anything I could think of. Of Mrs. Rose I got some Opium & a few ounces of garden peppers. I started back with a lightened heart. It was just dark as I got back. Mr. Galphin met me a few steps from the house. "You must prepare yourself for bad news, Allen," he said. I heard strange voices in the cabin, and I thought that either Dr. Daggert, or some physician travelling across the plains had come on to the Canon & had been sent up by the miners below, (as Hosea was thought a great deal of) and that it might have been pronounced necessary to amputate the foot. I was quite unprepared for the answer to 'my', "What it is?" "Hosea is dead!" Oh the terrible force of that blow! Oh! The utter desolation of that hour....

Truly and Affectionately your son

[Signed E. A. Grosh]

EDITORS' NOTE:

Reference: The original letter is in the possession of Charles T. Wegman of Bloomfield, New Jersey. His great-grandfather was Warren Rhinehart Grosh, a brother of Hosea and Ethan Grosh. A typed copy sent to Eric Moody of the Nevada Historical Society is used with Mr. Wegman's approval.

Vol. VIII, No. 3, Fall 1997

1887 TREATMENT
FOR 'BONE MARROW INFECTION'

Anton P. Sohn MD

Dr. John William Gunn graduated from Cooper Medical School in San Francisco and registered with the Lander County Recorder's Office in 1886 to practice in the area. In the described situation he treated a young man who had a compound fracture (bones protruding though the skin) of the lower extremity after falling off a horse. From the letter, Dr. Gunn was treating him for a bone marrow infection (osteomyelitis). The letter from Brotherton in Belmont to Dr. Gunn in Austin took two days. Gunn responded with the following letter and prescription. The Roberts state that Rhonan survived the injury.

DR. GUNN'S LETTER

Austin Nev. May 29/87

F. R. Brotherton Esq.
Belmont

Dear Sir.

Yours of 27th to hand and noted. From your description of Rhonans condition should say without a doubt, he has blood poison.

Symptoms ought to be besides pain you describe. Pulse 100 or more. Fever Resp. 20 to 40. Coated tongue bowels loose. Chill sweats Sweet breath perhaps cough and stained sputa.

Delirium, you say he has stupor. Bad signs are accumulation on teeth and gums, jerking, picking bed cloths etc. Some of these symptoms with be present. Chances are very much against recovery. Longer you can keep him alive, better.

Treatment – nothing special. If constipated and tongue coated five grs.

1. Blue Mass followed by magnesia in six hrs. Do not give if bowels loose. Give five grs. quinine every three hours with this or at intervals of four hrs. twenty drops Tinch. Iron

in water. If diarrhea is present do not try to check until it becomes exhaustive. Then use twenty drops of Laudanum with one oz. of Tr. Catechu & Chalk.

2. If pain severe ten gr. Dover powder or 1/6 gr. Morph. Repeated in two to six hours as required, If very weak may give five grs. of Ammonia Carbonate in milk every two–four hrs.

3. If cough troublesome ½ oz. of syr. sugar with the Ammonium. Besides the Quinine the most necessary is following. Whisky two oz. Milk twelve oz. Lime water eight oz.

4. Mix and give ¼ every hr. or two. Day and night. This is more important than medicine. May change off to wine and beef tea etc.

5. Locally to wound. Apply solution of 7½ grs. Corrosive Sublimate to pint of water or 1½ oz. Permanganate Potash to pint.

6. This is all you can do for him and probably this will not change result. As most all cases die.

7. You can let Ball and Deady read this, and you can get medicine as occasionally requires.

8. Probably trouble began from inflammation of marrow of leg bones. Pains in bones and joints are quite characteristic. You will probably find that his water contains a little albumin. Enclose Rx for iron and quinine.

Yours truly *JW Gunn*

Will send bill during week. Cannot get it sworn until after Memorial Day. *Dr. G.* Give him opiates enough to control pain. May take longer than I have ordered. *Dr. G.*

EDITORS' NOTE:

- In 2014, Allen and Karen Roberts of Fallon sent a copy of page 162 four-page handwritten letter to the editors detailing Dr. Gunn's instructions on how to treat Rhonan in 1887. Allen is the great grandson of 'Nellie' Goldbach, who was helping Rhonan's father, Frank Brotherton, care for his children. The Goldbachs homesteaded the Barley Creek Ranch in Monitor Valley.

- **Dover Powder** is a traditional medicine that was developed by Thomas Dover, an 18th-century British physician, for colds and fever. It contained ipecac, opium, lactose, and morphine.

- **Blue Mass (also known as calomel)** was a widely used 19th-century medicine that contained mercury chloride (a toxic substance that is a powerful acid and disinfectant) and blue chalk. President Lincoln used it for 'unknown reasons.'

- **Catechu** is an extract of the acacia tree and is an astringent that was frequently used in the 1800s.

- **Magnesia** is an ingredient of Milk of Magnesium and is a laxative and antacid.

- **Quinine**, an extract from the bark of the Peruvian Cinchona tree, has an interesting history. It has been used for hundreds of years to successfully eliminate the fever and chills of malaria by killing the organism, but it was not effective to treat any other cause of fever and chills. Malaria was prevalent in the Sacramento Delta and brought to Nevada by miners. In most cases quinine was efficacious if malaria was the cause. Unfortunately, malaria was not the cause of Rhonan's fever and chills. In addition, quinine was expensive and not always available. The editors maintain that quinine will cure what ails you if used with ice, gin, and a slice of lime in a drink known as gin and tonic.

Vol. XXV, No. 1, Spring 2014

GREAT BASIN SOLDIERS
COMSTOCK DISEASES

Anton P. Sohn MD

During the years of military presence in the Intermountain West, 1861-'65 (Civil War Years) servicemen in the East had a higher mortality and morbidity rate from disease than soldiers and male civilians in the West. The health conditions in the East reflected inadequate sanitation, poor hygiene due to crowding, and poor conditions during the Civil War. In the West, living conditions were more healthful due to less contamination of the environment and good climate.

Later, military surgeons commented on the salubrious effect of the climate and altitude on the health of the command. For instance, Surgeon Edward P. Vollum at Fort Douglas, Utah, in 1874 noted that he and the local physicians observed the beneficial effect of Utah's climate on phthisis (tuberculosis) and asthma. In a report to the Surgeon General, Vollum stated that there were no cases of phthisis that are "unconnected with heredity transmission." Furthermore, early cases of tuberculosis "get well spontaneously from the beneficial effects of the altitude and the inland dry character of the atmosphere." He continued, "The beneficial influence of this climate on asthma is decided and deserves a prominent mention."

On the other side of the Great Basin similar comments were made. In June 1867 at Fort Independence, California, Assistant Surgeon Washington Matthews stated that there was "one trifling case on sick-report during the month." In 1873, at Fort Warner, Oregon, there were three to six on sick report a month and an average strength of fifty men. In all, most soldiers enjoyed good health at the Great Basin commands.

Sanitation, hygiene, and adequate food supplies were still a problem for the soldiers stationed there. Doctors did not understand the role of the mosquito in malaria and the role of fomites (fomites are objects or materials that can carry disease) the spread of disease had not been elucidated.

As a result, food, water and utensils were sometimes contaminated; bad habits extended and increased the risk. In this environment epidemics of dysentery or diarrhea caused by cholera, typhoid and other enteric diseases were a threat to military camps and the civilian population.

Other diseases such as rheumatic fever spread in epidemic proportions through the West partly because the importance of the "contagious" sore throat was not associated with the severe arthritis. Frequent questions on the military examination for doctors emphasized concern about these issues. Thus, poor hygiene, uncleanliness and spread of contaminated material were the most important factors in the spread of infectious diarrhea, the most prevalent disorder on the frontier.

After diarrhea and other epidemic diseases the surgeon spent most of his time treating more mundane problems. By reviewing the hospital records one can get an idea of the day-to-day practice at Forts Churchill, Bidwell (California), Halleck, Independence (California), McDermit and other Great Basin posts. During 1860 and 1861 the aggregate strength of Fort Churchill varied from 182 to 284 while admissions to the hospital varied from twenty-three to seventy per month. During one month an outbreak of diarrhea and other diseases hospitalized 34 percent of the command, with an average length of stay of three days, leaving no doubt that the hospital was full, and the strength of the command was depleted.

Between 1870 and 1874, health conditions at seven Great Basin forts–Cameron (Utah), Bidwell, Douglas (Utah), Halleck, Harney (Oregon), Independence and McDermit–were reported to the Surgeon General. At Fort Cameron the mean strength of the command varied between 181 and 215 men and upper respiratory infections led the list with eleven cases.

Although respiratory infections were, from time to time, a problem in the Great Basin, diarrhea was a greater threat to life. Fort Douglas had an average of 364 men and diarrhea was the most common disease with 836 cases over a four-year period.

Trauma from accidents with 671 cases, malarial fever with 472 and rheumatism with 400 were next in frequency. Later in the 1890s when 600 were stationed at Fort Douglas, Assistant Surgeon Deshon reported: "The hospital averaged about twenty patients, with tonsillitis, rheumatic affections, venereal disease and trauma being most common."

At Fort Halleck with a mean strength of ninety-nine men and four to six officers, the most common cause for sick call was trauma (152 cases during the same period). Harney had mean strength of fifty-six and trauma was also the most common disorder with 176 cases. Independence had a mean strength of forty-eight to sixty-six and rheumatism and accidents were equal with forty cases each. At McDermit the mean strength was fifty-nine men with two to three officers and fever led the list with 103 cases. No fort was immune to alcoholism, intestinal disorders and other disease that occurred.

Over the four-year period there were 1,477 men per year on sick call (not including trauma) at the seven bases (Cameron, Bidwell, Douglas, Halleck, Harney, Independence and McDermit). The average number of men stationed at these combined bases was approximately 969 producing a sick rate of 1,524 per 1,000 men. During this period the sick rate for the whole United States Army varied from a high of 2,087 in 1871 to a low of 1,561 in 1873. Therefore, the military sick rate on the Great Basin appeared to be at the low end of the average for the Army. the rate is 1,824 per 1,000 men.

A further breakdown of the specific illnesses during this early period reveals diarrhea accounting for 18.4 percent of the cases, trauma accounted for 18.2 percent of the cases, malarial fevers were 12.1 percent and rheumatism resulted in 9.5 percent of the entries. Alcoholism accounted for a high percentage of the admissions, overall it was 3.6 percent. Another social problem among soldiers was venereal disease. It was less than one half as prevalent as alcoholism. In an interesting observation, Dr. Kober, in unpublished memoirs from Fort Bidwell estimated that as high as fifty percent of the soldiers who reported for sick call would not have complained in civilian life.

A word of caution is necessary about prevalence of disease in the nineteenth century because some diseases were confused with others. The diarrhea seen with scurvy was confused with the diarrhea of gastrointestinal disease. Scurvy associated arthritis was confused with other causes of joint pain and stiffness of the lower extremities. Also, fever and malaise associated with many infectious diseases sometimes overshadowed the more diagnostic features resulting in misdiagnosis. Thus, malaria in camps during the Spanish-American War of 1898 was often confused with typhoid fever. The differences in criteria for diagnosis were significant.

Vol. V, No. 4, Winter 1994-5

SOLDIERS' DIAGNOSES
FORT CHURCHILL'S HOSPITAL
Personnel at the Fort—207 to 198 soldiers
Date of Admissions—July 1860 to January 1862

Disease	Totals	%
Intermittent fever	121	18.3
Diarrhea	77	11.6
Rheumatism	72	10.9
Trauma	67	10.2
Catarrh	60	9.1
Tonsillitis	25	3.8
Ophthalmia	20	3.0
Digestive complaints	20	3.0
Constipation	19	2.9
Neuralgia	18	2.7
Syphilis	18	2.7
Gonorrhea	14	2.1
Bronchitis	13	2.0
Subcutaneous abscess	11	1.7
Paronychia	9	1.4
Delirium tremens	9	1.4
Hepatitis	8	1.2
Hemorrhoids	6	0.9
Pleuritis	5	0.8
Otitis	4	0.6
Toothache	4	0.6
Lumbago	3	0.5
Orchitis	3	0.5
Pneumonia	2	0.3
Scrofula	1	0.2
Scorbutus	1	0.2
Other	50	7.6
Totals	660	100.0%

SAINT MARY LOUISE PATIENTS DIAGNOSES
March 1876 to Dec. 1877

Disease	Totals	%
Typhoid/typhus	54	18.2
Trauma	51	17.2
Fevers (all)	31	10.4
Abscess/inflame	23	7.7
Nervous debility	22	7.4
Consumption	18	6.1
Pneumonia	14	4.7
Rheumatism	13	4.4
Diarrhea	10	3.4
Erysipelas	8	2.7
Nervous sys. disease	8	2.7
Salivated (syphilis)	8	2.7
Digestive complaints	5	1.7
Liver disease	4	1.3
Burns	4	1.3
Sore leg/finger/arm	4	1.3
Delirium tremens	3	1.0
Amputation	3	1.0
Ophthalmia	3	1.0
Insanity	2	1.0
Enlarged veins	1	0.7
Bronchitis	1	0.7
Pleuritis	1	0.7
Diphtheria	1	0.7
Cancer/throat	1	0.7
Asthma	1	0.7
Cramps	1	0.7
Dropsy	1	0.7
Anal fistula	1	0.7
Totals	297	100%

It is difficult to compare diagnosis of frontier soldiers to miners and citizens on the Comstock because of differences in age, sex, unregulated physicians, and other unknown characteristics, but there are some similarities. Intermittent fever (malaria) was the most common diagnosis at Fort Churchill's Hospital, and fevers, including malaria, were the third most common diagnosis on the Comstock. As might be expected, trauma was high on the list at Saint Mary Louise Hospital due to accidents in a mining community. On occasion, trauma topped the list of diagnoses at Nevada's forts.

During the time period covered by the above statistics. Death from trauma—if not the event—the infections that was likely to occur was twice as likely as in 2014. Not only was emergency help not available, treatment and surgery were not developed to handle the complications of hemorrhage and nonunion of the bones.

CHAPTER VII:
NINETEENTH-CENTURY DOCTORS

This story began in 1851 when Doctors Charles Daggett and T.A. Hylton appeared in Mormon Station. Nothing is known about Hylton, but Daggett, who was also an attorney, played a prominent part in Nevada becoming a state. He also made medical history when he treated Orson Hyde's frozen feet in 1855, thereby recording the first know treatment of a patient in what would become Nevada. What is remarkable is that he gave the right therapy in spite of the fact that medicine in mid-19th century was primitive when compared to today.

Before microbial cause of disease was discovered in the late 1880s, medical treatment was little more than home remedy. For example, in 1868 smallpox treatment by Dr. Zabriske was by, "…good grub, keep your bowels in order, use a reasonable amount of choice whiskey, gin, brandy–whichever you prefer–and keep out of the way of the disease as much as possible." Today, we know that the last part of this statement was his only good advice.

Mining towns in the 1900s had ineffective sewerage systems. In 1875 'earthy matter,' or human waste, polluting drinking water was the cause of disease at Fort McDermit, which is located in Nevada at the Oregon border. Water contamination, infectious diseases such as tuberculosis, scarlet fever, typhoid fever, and diphtheria were leading causes of death in the 1880s. During this time u.s. life expectancy at birth was less than forty years, but it steadily increased over the next one hundred years. Not only were these improvements due to the recognition of the importance of sterility and avoiding harmful organisms, but they were due to advances in diagnosis and treatment of disease and changes in diet.

NEVADA'S FIRST DOCTOR
DR. CHARLES DAGGETT

Ryan Davis, History Student

On a bleak night in December 1855, Judge Orson Hyde (1805-1878), a well-known Mormon traveler and missionary, was expecting to die in the mountains. His hope of crossing the Sierra Nevada into the Carson City area was quickly fading before his eyes. With unparalleled will he managed to trudge on, rolling down snowy inclines, finding his way to the cabin of Dr. Charles Daggett.

Daggett had settled in a log cabin situated at the base of the Georgetown cut-off on the emigrant trail. Because of his prestige in the little community, it took on his name and became known as Daggett Pass.

Dogs outside of Daggett's house alerted him to the presence of a visitor, and he found the exhausted shell of Hyde. Seeing frozen feet, Daggett did not bring the man into the warmth of the cabin but took him to a frozen stream, chopped a hole into the ice, and urged the weary traveler to dangle his black board-like swollen legs and feet into the icy water. Once the legs began to feel soft to the touch Daggett helped Hyde into his home where he rubbed the thawed limbs with turpentine and packed them in fluffy raw cotton.

As simple as the entire ordeal may seem today, Dr. Daggett and Mr. Hyde were unaware at the time that this act was to become one of the first documented cases of medical treatment in what would become the state of Nevada. It was one in a string of firsts which Dr. Daggett would take part in, throughout the remainder of his life in Nevada. Not only is the case remarkable in that it is the first known medical treatment in what is now Nevada, but it also is a textbook example of how frostbite is treated in similar circumstances today. The treatment of frostbite is a process of gradual warming rather than sudden heat application.

In fact, over one hundred years ago Russian fishermen knew that sudden warming of frozen fish resulted in mushy flesh, while slowly warming the flesh resulted in firmer more normal meat. What is remarkable is that a doctor who lived over 150 years ago was able to apply the best medical knowledge to treat frozen feet in that manner.

Born in Vermont in 1806, Charles Daggett graduated from the Berkshire Medical College in Massachusetts, where he also received a law degree. In 1851, he moved west with a man known only by the name of Gay, settling in the area then known as Mormon Station, a few miles from Genoa. Daggett and his companion settled in the log cabin Hyde stumbled upon shortly after their move to Mormon Station. Kingsbury Road, where the cabin was located, was a trail that had been established shortly before Daggett moved to the community.

Dr. Daggett was selected as prosecuting attorney, county assessor, and tax collector of Carson County on September 20, 1855. Daggett not being a member of the lds faith enhanced his value to Orson Hyde as the tax collector. People in Carson Valley had never paid taxes before and were outraged. Dr. Daggett's life was openly threatened over this. Because of the reluctance of the locals to come under 'Mormon Law' almost everyone on the first 'Mormon Ticket' was a non-Mormon. Dr. Daggett became Nevada's first 'resident' attorney on November 2, 1855, just hours before he tried his first case. The first attorney in the territory that would become Nevada was Col. L.A. Norton, a 'temporary' resident from Placerville.

One of his last known distinctions occurred when he was appointed a member of the Committee of Arrangements for the formation of the Second Convention to form a separate territory out of the Utah Territory. With Dr. Daggett's persistence, this territory became the State of Nevada. After his political career he settled in the Genoa area and there is no official surviving document attesting to the year or his age when he died.

EDITORS' NOTE:

Guy Rocha supplied the source, and Robert Ellison of the Nevada Library and Archives supplied information for this article.

Vol. XIV, No. 3, Fall 2003

ADDENDUM TO
Dr. Daggett's Treatment

Letter from Orson Hyde to Brigham Young, Genoa, Jan. 13, 1856.

> Next morning made a sure course and after two days hard tracking got in to Dr. Daggett's House and limbs much swollen, feet like marbles, tired completely out four nights without sleep on half rations—spent and sagging, marred and shattered, but back sound and good. Put feet and legs into cold water. Then turpentine and raw cotton. Next morning came home in a buggy. One foot now well, the other doing well, but looks as much like anything other than a foot. Doct. Says he think will only lose my little toe on the right root. I fell first rate have only lost 50 pounds of flesh with the freeze and pain. Labour is a quiet relief and amusement to me. When my foot gets well I think that I shall be all right….

Letter from Orson Hyde to Brigham Young, Genoa, Jan. 25, 1856.

> Frozen feet cause hand to tremble, so you must excuse. I believe the head is steady and unquivering.
>
> An Indian is doctoring my feet. He says No Walk—No smoke—No drink fire water, but sit still and do as he says, and in some manner (Ten days) feet be heap goddie….

EDITORS' NOTE:

Robert Ellison of the Nevada Library and Archives supplied copies of the letters from Hyde to Young.

ZABRISKE'S DISINFECTANT
Dr. Christian Zabriske

Anton P. Sohn MD

Dr. Christian Bevoort Zabriske was no ordinary Polish descendent born in the usa; he had a dream to explore the unknown and help others overcome illness. He was born in Haversack, New Jersey, on June 29, 1801, into a family that had emigrated from Poland in the 1660s. He received an MD from Columbia University in 1832; however, his vision led him west. He and son Elias moved to Jacksonville, Illinois, where he joined as a volunteer for the Mexican War in 1846. After the war he was back in New York as a surgeon for the California Union Association that had plans to go to the California goldfields.

Initially landing in Panama with his fellow passengers, he found over 2,000 other travelers stranded and waiting for passage to California. The group raised $6,000, bought a dilapidated schooner, and sailed up the coast to San Francisco. His brother, James, remained in California to practice law while Dr. Zabriske and son continued to Silver City, Nevada Territory.

The 1862 Directory lists Dr. Zabriske as living on Second Street between High and Main with son Elias, an attorney. Various directories and advertisements during the 1860s and 1870s list seven additional doctors living or practicing in Silver City.

His patient ledgers start October 12, 1862, and show appointments through October 4, 1868. Many of the notations were after midnight. Irene Brennan's article in the August 17, 1975, *Review Journal*'s *Nevadan* notes that Zabriske's fees ranged from $2 to $10, but his collections were about 30 percent. For example, during September 1863 his charges were $1,013.50 and payments were $368. Brennan further notes, "By Cash (Greenbacks) $70.00." To further add to his collection deficit woes, Greenbacks sold at the local banks for between 68¢ and 72¢ on the dollar.

Zabriske's ledgers give some insight into this practice. He used the lancet, as was the practice at the time, to bleed patients. In addition, he used blistering, scarification, and cupping. Blistering was a procedure when blisters were produced by applying burning heat and lancing the blisters to drain fluid. Scarification resulted when a flat surfaced gadget with six or eight spring-loaded lancets pierced the skin or mucous membrane to produce oozing of blood or serum. To increase oozing a heated glass cup was placed over the wounds to create suction.

Dr. Zabriske charged $50 for a delivery and on one occasion he charged $15 for delivering a placenta. Smallpox was a threat to 19th-century citizens of Nevada, and the doctor charged Lyon County for treating the illness. He also vaccinated patients to prevent the dreaded disease. The following was in the *Gold Hill Daily News* 12/11/1868: Zabriske's Disinfectant—Speaking of Chloride of lime, carbolic acid and other popular disinfectants, Dr. Zabriske says the best way to fortify against the smallpox is to eat plenty of good grub, keep your bowels in order, use a reasonable amount of choice whiskey, gin, brandy—whichever you prefer—and keep out of the way of the disease as much as possible. The Doctor's head is pretty level, but what's a poor fellow like us to do who hasn't got any mouth for whiskey?

There was professional courtesy among doctors in Silver City. Zabriske and Dr. Sheldon McMeans amputated a badly broken leg after teamster Ezekiel W. Culliver splintered his leg in two places. On another occasion Dr. Zabriske set Joseph Todman's broken femur and charged $50. He consulted with Dr. Minneer regarding Todman and after seven visits found it necessary to perform a "bleeding." He sometimes used a starch bandage to immobilize a fracture. His ledger showed that he charged $50 for syphilis treatment. He treated fourteen cases of syphilis (three were secondary syphilis) and eight cases of gonorrhea.

Dr. Christian Zabriske died at the Reno Asylum November 1886, and Candelaria's *True Fissure* noted in an obituary: Dr. Zabriske… represented Lyon Co. in Republican conventions many times. An able physician, possessed of a gigantic brain, one of the handsomest men the writer ever saw.

IMPORTANT PIONEER DOCTOR
DR. HENRY BERGSTEIN

Henry Bergstein was born in Virginia in 1847 to German speaking Jewish parents. At an early age, he came west and enrolled in the Medical College of the Pacific in San Francisco, where he graduated in 1872. Dr. Samuel Cooper founded the school in 1858. In 1882, it became Cooper Medical College, and in 1912, Stanford Medical School. The same year he graduated he moved to Pioche, Nevada, where he was instrumental in forming an association of physicians. It appears that the primary reason for their meeting was to set or control fees. Some of the fees they agreed upon were as follows: office visits $5, night visits $10, delivery $100, and operations $100 and up.

Bergstein astutely observed that most Pioche citizens died from accidents, gunshot wounds, and knife injuries. He noted that of 108 "denizens" in the local graveyard, only three died of natural causes. He was even more alarmed that a local druggist treated miners with quicksilver (mercury) when they presented with constipation due to lead poisoning. The druggist "succeeded in giving them a passage to the grave." At that time there were no licensing laws in Nevada, and because of an "everyman is his own doctor attitude," few had been passed in the rest of the nation. To remedy the situation, Bergstein ran for the legislature in 1874. After election he moved to Virginia City in 1875 with the intent of initiating legislation to limit the practice of medicine to qualified persons.

His law had several sections, but most importantly, it required doctors to have it recorded with the county recorder.

Not only did Nevada not have a method to verify the diplomas, but also there were no uniform requirements for medical schools in the U.S. Anyone could start a medical school and issue a diploma. Furthermore, many doctors graduated from foreign schools, which could not be verified. This included a plethora of Chinese doctors with diplomas written in Chinese script. Governor L.R. Bradley forced through a ten-year grandfather clause that permitted unqualified doctors to continue practice.

Doctors Bergstein, John W. Vanzant, and Benjamin Robinson were the leaders in forming the Nevada State Medical Society, which enforced the new law. The law was short lived, as it was later declared unconstitutional by the Nevada Supreme Court.

Medical practice aside, in 1880, Bergstein married Pauline Michelson in San Francisco.

Later that year he became entangled in a law suit with D.L. Brown, editor of *Footlight*, a Nevada newspaper, for an article that Bergstein claimed was derogatory to him as physician. The case was dropped, but Bergstein continued to be controversial. In 1883, he was associated with Dr. Simeon Bishop, the second superintendent of the Nevada Hospital for Indigent Insane in Sparks. He accused Bishop of misappropriation of funds.

On the political side, Dr. Bergstein was lifelong member of the Democratic Party, but in 1892 he stepped down as chairman of the Washoe County Democrat Party to join the Silver Party.

Bergstein was instrumental in reestablishing nsma in 1894. As a result he was elected president of the society and state delegate to the ama. After 1895 the state society met regularly, and members presented scientific papers. Bergstein's contribution was a paper in 1912 on "Criminal Abortion from a Moral and Business Standpoint."

His next controversial episode resulted after he succeeded Dr. Simeon Bishop as superintendent of The Hospital for Indigent Insane in Sparks. Bergstein held this position from 1895 until 1898, when his term of office expired. Psychiatry was in its infancy, but Dr. Bergstein was in the forefront of humane care for the mentally ill.

He stopped the "custom of placing the inmates on exhibit for the amusement of and to gratify the morbid curiosity of visitors," and he changed the name to Nevada Hospital for Mental Disease. Bergstein would have been held in high esteem for these actions, but his feisty nature continued to get him in trouble.

In 1897, Bergstein fired his business manager, who retaliated by charging him with "performing unauthorized autopsies on patients, then throwing parts of their bodies in the nearby Truckee River." At a hearing of the State Mental Hospital Commission, "Bergstein defended himself by arguing that the patients were deceased and without families, [sic] what he did with their bodies made no difference." It appears from witnesses and by his statement that he disposed of human remains, including brain tissue, in the Truckee, but the Board of Commissioners dismissed the charges.

By this time, his domestic life was becoming chaotic. He "deserted and abandoned" Pauline and divorced her two years later. She was to receive $100/month for support of their three children and a dwelling at 2nd and Chestnut (Arlington) in Reno, which is now the site of St. Thomas Aquinas Cathedral. Court fights between the two would continue for years and were remarkable for Bergstein's lack of paying.

Bergstein was unable to establish a successful practice in Reno after his 1900 marriage to Clara Poor Powning, widow of prominent Reno citizen C.C. Powning, so the couple moved to San Francisco. In spite of the move, financial problems continue to plague Henry. In 1907 hotelier J.M. McCormack seized his surgical instruments (worth $275) for an unpaid bill. By this time he was separated from Clara, and he described himself as "...an old and broken man, with his earning capacity very much limited, and without any resources except his practice…." He also noted that his 3 sons had assumed the name Michelson, his ex-wife's maiden name. That year, her brother, Albert, received the Nobel Prize for Physics. Apparently Henry was paying some alimony, but Pauline accused him of being "addicted to gambling" resulted in his inability to pay support.

By 1908, Bergstein was practicing again in Reno, and the 1910 census listed him as widowed. His private life difficulties apparently had not damaged his professional reputation, and he became prominent in Nevada's medical circles. His responsibilities included Reno City Physician, Reno City Health Inspector, and member of the Reno City Board of Health. Henry's knowledge and position in the medical community prompted Sam P. Davis to ask him to write Nevada Medical History for *The History of Nevada*, which Davis published in 1913.

In 1920, Doctor Henry Bergstein was practicing at 117 North Virginia, but in 1921, there is no mention of him in the City Telephone directory. Apparently he died in 1920 or 1921, but there is no record of his death in Nevada vital statistics.

EDITORS' NOTE:

Information in this article is taken from UNR Professor John P. Marschall's research for a book he is writing on a comprehensive history of Jews in Nevada. According to Dr. Marschall: "No physician in Nevada's early history was more influential than Henry Bergstein. His years of service to the state as a physician, legislator, organizer, and superintendent of the State Mental Hospital spanned the period from 1872 beyond 1920. Although he had left the state briefly in 1900 upon his second marriage to the widow of his political associate, C.C. Powning, he returned to Reno where he struggled to make a living. Sam Davis called upon Bergstein to contribute to Davis' forthcoming book, History of Nevada, with an essay on the history of medicine in the state. Bergstein was a natural choice for the project in view of his long tenure as a physician and his administrative responsibilities.

Vol. II, No. 2, Summer 1991

Vol. XVII, No. 3, Winter 2007

HYDROPATHIC MEDICINE
DOCTORS ADA AND GIDEON WEED

Kristin Sohn, UNSOM Student

Doctors Gideon A. and Ada M. Weed brought eastern hydropathic medicine to the western frontier in 1858. The couple met while enrolled in Dr. Russell T. Trall's Hygeio-Therapeutic College in New York City. In 1857, they both received 'irregular diplomas,' as the institution did not yet have a charter. Dr. Trall's college taught the principles of hydrotherapy, also known as the 'water-cure,' which was considered an alternative to allopathic medicine. Supporters believed that drug therapies were unnecessary and, in fact, detrimental to successful medical treatment. Instead, practitioners of hydrotherapy relied on principles of hygiene, diet, rest, and the therapeutic value of water.

Dr. Trall established hydrotherapy as a medical system in the United States during the 1840s. Admission requirements to his school included a 'common school education and the possession of common sense.' Most students were from the working class, and he advocated training women, despite the societal restrictions of the time. In fact, a third of Trall's graduates were female, during a time when it was extremely difficult for women to gain admission into traditional medical schools.

A few months after graduation Ada (1837-1910) and Gideon (1833-1905) were married in the school's lecture hall. The couple quickly departed the east coast for the western frontier; they arrived in San Francisco in early 1858. Unlike many who migrated during this time, the Weeds did not plan to make a quick fortune and return east; they actually planned to settle in California and make a home there. They dreamed of opening their own Hygeio-Medical Institute. Unfortunately, unforeseen professional competition existed in San Francisco, and the Weeds decided to continue their migration into Oregon.

Oregon proved to be a state with abundant opportunities for the Weeds. The territory lacked hydropathic physicians, and, furthermore, there existed a great demand for their services. Readers had actually written to the editor of *The Water Cure Journal*, asking for both a hydropathic physician and a hydropathic institution in their area. The Weeds rented an office in Salem and advertised in the *Oregon Statesman*. They began plans for a water cure establishment, which would include bathing facilities, a gymnasium, and boarding rooms. Ida focused on the female populations, advertising a specialty in obstetrics and pediatrics.

Soon after their arrival, the Weeds began eliciting criticism and stirring controversy. Being 'irregular practitioners,' they were subjected to criticism by those who believed in traditional medicine. The women mistrusted Ida because she was the first female in Oregon with a medical degree. The couple was also suspect because they actively advertised. Lastly, the couple stirred controversy because they advocated social change. In addition to curing people of their ills, they desired to cure society of its problems.

Ida, in particular, strongly pushed for social reform. She gave a series of lectures to Oregonians, in which she espoused woman's rights and the need for improved conditions among frontier women. Although her efforts produced no significant changes or advancements among women in Oregon, she did succeed in eliciting controversy and gaining opposition. Perhaps her strongest and most publicized opposition was from Asahel Bush, editor of the *Oregon Statesmen*. After hearing one of Ida's first lectures, he published several lengthy critiques in his newspaper. Ida issued rebuttals, but her reputation had been permanently damaged.

The Weeds continued their reform efforts despite this opposition. They traveled among various settlements in the Oregon region, and gave talks in churches and courtrooms. Some lectures were free, and others required a 50¢ admission fee. Most likely to avoid male criticism, such as that she had received from Asahel Bush, Ida often gave lectures to female only crowds. Her topics expanded to sex and birth control.

Portions of the public soon began to view her as a woman's rights zealot.

Despite the negative publicity the Weeds outwardly painted their crusade as successful. They believed they were making headway in converting the public towards hydrotherapy. In correspondence with Dr. Trall, they claimed that the people of Oregon were in a 'transitional state' and opposed traditional medicine and its drugs, but did not yet fully support hydrotherapy. Additionally, they believed that the traditional doctors in Oregon, who initially denounced hydrotherapy, were beginning to claim that they had always used water therapy in their treatments.

After their second lecture tour they wrote accounts of receptive audiences, many of whom were already practicing their principles. They described the success of their practice, and claimed they had as many patients as their house could hold. They failed, however, to divulge their financial hardships. As the economy in Oregon was depressed, many patients were unable to pay. The Weeds took on a partner to help finance the outfitting of their treatment house. Their lectures were well attended, their profits did not cover expenses.

Unable to get ahead in Oregon, the Weeds returned to California in the spring of 1860. A year later they opened a Hygeio-Medical Institute in Sacramento. Even though this was their unfulfilled dream while in Oregon, the Weeds were still unable to settle down and prosper. That fall they followed the silver rush to Washoe City, Nevada where Gideon became successful. They returned again to California, settling in Vallejo. It seems that they remained restless.

In 1869, at the age of thirty-six Gideon returned to school and received eighteen weeks of allopathic training at Rush Medical College in Chicago. This marked a turning point for the couple, as their success and status greatly improved, and they were no longer met with strong opposition. In 1870 they moved to Seattle, where Gideon practiced as a physician and surgeon. He enjoyed a lucrative practice and refocused his reform energies on improving healthcare conditions.

In 1874, Gideon founded the Seattle Hospital to improve medical care for those injured in the logging camps and saw mills around the area. He provided medical care to indigent, was active in various medical societies, assisted in creating the State Medical Board, and helped secure funds to start a medical school. During 2 terms as mayor, he was able to pass many reforms and earn respect from fellow citizens. In fact, he was the 1st mayor to succeed at reelection.

Mrs. Weed did not continue to practice medicine after their move to Seattle. Furthermore, neither Doctors Weed advertised their hydropathic degrees or continued lecturing. Gideon's medical practice, along with wise real estate investments, allowed the couple to maintain a high quality of life. They built a mansion in 1876 and raised two children, Benjamin and Mabel. Ada became somewhat of a society lady. She hosted social events at their mansion, served as director of the Library Association, represented the Plymouth Congregational Church, and supported charities. She continued to push for women's rights, but she allied with the local temperance movement and shunned the more dramatic suffragists. Additionally, she assisted her husband in his medical reform activities.

While in Seattle, the Weeds were very successful in their medical and social reform activities. Their newfound traditional methods were in stark contrast to the previous methods they had utilized while in Oregon and California. They garnered significant respect from the citizens of Washington, and they avoided the criticism and opposition they had received during previous crusades. A detailed article ran in Seattle's *Pacific Tribune* on October 25, 1877, which described their twentieth wedding anniversary. They received valuable China pieces as gifts from other prominent citizens, which testified to their important position in their community.

In 1890,the Weeds moved to Berkeley, where Gideon continued to practice traditional medicine and the children attended the University of California. The couple's nephew, Dr. Park Weed Willis, an allopathic physician trained at the University of Pennsylvania, took over Gideon's Seattle medical practice.

Ada continued to be active in social causes, and she assisted victims of the San Francisco earthquake. In her final years, she nursed her paralytic husband and continued to practice her hydropathic beliefs. She suffered from a variety of physical ailments and continued to drink large amounts of water, self-treatment of which her nephew approved. She died of cancer in 1910.

EDITORS' NOTE:

Reference: Thomas G. Edwards, "Dr. Ada M. Weed: Northwest Reformer," (*Oregon Historical Quarterly*, 1978, 1).

Vol. XIX, No. 3, Fall 2008

Vol. XX, No. 1, Spring 2009

ADVENTURES OF DR. ANTON TJADER

San Francisco Herald September 9, 1859, by correspondent 'Tennessee' Richard Allen, from Genoa, Carson Valley, Utah Territory: "Dr. A.W. Tjader, a Russian gentleman now sojourning here, is the one who took care of the wounded immigrants, survivors of the late Indian massacre on the Sublette Cutoff. He performed this kindness without reward or the hope of reward; and is, in my opinion, justly entitled to public gratitude. I am in hopes that he will remain with us and practice his profession".

There is some question with regard to the birthplace of Dr. Anton W. Tjader. Despite his Swedish name, he described himself as Russian and the headstone on his grave lists his birthplace as St. Petersburg, Russia, 1825. His great grandson, however, claimed that he had verification of Anton's birth and registration in Stockholm, Sweden, in 1827. Anton Tjader received his MD degree from the Royal Scandinavia Institute in Uppsala, Sweden, and served as a surgeon in the Russian Army during the Crimean Wars of 1854. After immigrating to the United States in 1855, he entered Harvard Medical School, graduated two years later, and served as a United States Army Contract Surgeon.

In 1859, Dr. Tjader joined the movement west, traveling with the Scroggs wagon train from Missouri. It was during this trek that Anton Tjader became involved with the Shepherd Train Massacre on the Sublette Cutoff.

William Shepherd, with the Shepherd Train, was traveling one day ahead of the Scroggs train when he became ill with mountain fever. On July 18, 1859, his brother James and another man backtracked the trail in search of a doctor. Dr. Tjader agreed to ride up and attend the sick man. Examining the patient the doctor determined that the man's fever had broken and pronounced him out of danger. The captain of the Shepherd Train, Ferguson Shepherd, was eager to press on, and by July 26, they had reached Cold Springs camp on the Sublette Cutoff and found the camp in a state of shock.

According to statements given when they reached Genoa a month later: "About 6:00 pm on July 26, when some men, of a small emigrant train camped at Cold Springs on the Sublette cutoff eighty miles from Salt Lake City, were at supper a small party of eight Indians arrived with rifles, bows and arrows came down and asked for something to eat. Having obtained some bread, they started to a hill where two men herded cattle. After saluting the cattle guards and passing them, one of the Indians suddenly turned his pony, lowering his rifle, shot one of the men, Mr. Hall, through the heart, killing him Instantly. The other-man fled to the camp. The Indians were in the meantime running off nine cattle and two horses."

Despite attempts to convince Capt. Ferguson Shepherd to remain in Cold Springs until they could assemble a larger train, he decided to continue on as a small train. The statement continues: At the time of the depredation there were only a small number of train emigrants present, and sometime afterward, at about 9:00 o'clock, the horse train led by Mr. Ferguson Shepherd arrived… in the morning, Mr. Shepherd's train left at 7:00 o'clock, at the arrival of the Skroggs Train in spite of the warnings of danger.

At 11:00 o'clock the train entered a narrow canyon seven miles from the Cold Springs camp. A horse, which had been sick, stopped and would go no further. The men gathered around the horse to discuss the situation. Distracted by the sick horse, their guard was down. Suddenly gunfire erupted. Captain Shepherd and two other men fell seriously wounded. Next, William Shepherd was shot in the shoulder, then in the forehead. He was the first to die. Uninjured men from the train began to shoot back. Some began running from the scene heading back toward the Cold Springs camp.

Annie Shepherd began to run with her baby, Ida, in her arms. Encumbered by her long dress and the baby, she soon became exhausted and grew faint. She asked Smith to carry Ida, but Smith had been shot in the arm above the elbow. The bone was broken, and he was losing blood. Soon he became exhausted and faint. Unable to continue with the baby, he set her down in a grove of poplar trees and covered her with grass and leaves. Near dark he lay down in some sagebrush unable to move on. Another man found him and took him back into the Cold Springs camp, where Dr. Tjader treated his wounds.

In the end Captain Ferguson Shepherd, his brother William, and two other men were dead. Five people were wounded. The Wrights, traveling with the Shepherds were both shot and stayed with the wagons in the canyon. Throughout the afternoon and evening people straggled back into Cold Springs. Annie stumbled into camp at sunset "in a state of insanity." Placed in a bed she immediately asked to see her baby. "She's in another wagon as requested by Dr. Tjader, and you are too exhausted to see her," said James Shepherd.

Annie pleaded with Dr. Tjader, and he finally relented the truth that Ida, just seven months old, was still out on the trail. "Annie raved like a maniac the entire night."

Two more wagon trains joined the party in Cold Springs camp that afternoon arid early the next morning the united trains with fifty-two wagons and two hundred men started through the canyon, led by a group of ten-armed men. As they reached the grove of poplar trees the men were heard shouting. The baby was found alive. Badly dehydrated and sunburned, the baby was barely alive when she was returned to a joyous Annie, who nursed the baby back to health with the help of Dr. Tjader.

...The bodies of Ferguson and William Shepherd, William Diggs, and C. Rains were found in the road, covered with blood, dead, and bloated by the heat, some twenty-four hours after the attack.

Upon reaching the wagons, the party found Mrs. James Wright lying under a wagon holding a crippled baby in her arms. Mrs. Wright had a serious wound in her back. Nearby lay mortally wounded James Wright, who died two days later. The poor sufferers had been attended by their little five-year-old son, who supplied their feverish lips with water.

The wagon train continued and reached Genoa on September 2, 1859. Dr. Tjader established a medical practice in that community, and then, he removed his practice to Carson City in 1860. On May 14, 1860, he volunteered for the Carson City Rangers and was involved in the Battle of Pyramid Lake. Although reported to have been killed and scalped, Dr Tjader returned from that skirmish with three slight arrow wounds and resumed his medical practice, which he continued until his death on July 8, 1870, at the age of forty-four.

EDITORS' NOTE:

The above story about Dr. Anton Tjader was carefully researched by his great grandson, Mr. Gary Tinder of Los Altos, California.

It represents only a small portion of the biographical material being assembled by Gary Tjader, who intends to publish the entire story at a later date. Our thanks to Mr. Tjader for allowing us to use this interesting look at the practice of medicine in the 19th century.

Vol. V, No. 3, Fall 1994

Vol. VII, No. 2, Summer 1996

DR. ANTON W. TJADER'S
CAREER IN NEVADA

In addition to his medical duties, Dr. Tjader performed community service and served as secretary at a citizens' meeting. The minutes of the various meetings in the community only name one doctor in town, Dr. Tjader. Nevertheless, his time in Genoa was short, and on April 14, 1860, he moved to Carson City. There he is noted to have 'gunshot wounds a specialty.' Thus he began a medical practice in his new home.

Also in 1860, a skirmish broke out at a trading post near the future site of Fort Churchill. Two young Indian girls were kidnapped, and when they were rescued, two white men were killed and one drowned while attempting to flee. A hastily assembled group of 105 men set out from the Carson/Virginia City area in May 1860 to punish the responsible Indians, who were camped near Pyramid Lake. The militia included three doctors, Tjader, William Eichelroth, and Rezin Bell. The party was overwhelmed and the leader, Colonel Ormsby was killed. Allen, again was impressed with Tjader's valor wrote, "Dr. Tjader, a gentleman of Russian birth, very highly esteemed here, not only on account of his skill as a surgeon and physician, but also because of his kind and amiable disposition, was reported killed and scalped. Several of those who were in the battle have told me that they saw him fall in the very midst of the enemy, but after five days' wandering, without food or shelter, he reached Virginia City last night, only slightly wounded." His survival was of heroic proportions and remains a legend to this day.

Later in November 1860, Dr. Tjader performed what may be the first autopsy in the territory on Jonathon Carr, who was hanged in its first execution. Doctors Munckton and Daggett pronounced Carr dead, and Tjader received $50 for the autopsy.

In 1862, Dr. Tjader helped newly arrived Dr. Charles L. Anderson establish a practice in the community. Dr. Tjader was appointed surgeon general of the Nevada Militia in 1864. One year later he married Lucy Curry, daughter of the Abe Curry, the founder of Carson City.

In a spoof of Nevada politics, Mark Twain in *Early Tales and Sketches* wrote the following of Dr. Tjader: "I will adjourn the convention for one hour, on account of my cold, to the end that I may apply the remedy prescribed by Dr. Tjader–the same being gin and molasses. The Chief Page is hereby instructed to provide a spoonful of molasses and a gallon of gin, for the use of the President."

For a short while in 1866 Tjader practiced in Washoe City, but he returned to Carson City in 1867. In 1870 Dr. Tjader died leaving two infant sons and a widow. The death notice in the paper stated: "A diseased state of both heart and lungs, these superinducing dropsy of the abdomen and lower extremities. He has been a great sufferer, but heroically patient and courageous. His demise was expected any time during the past few weeks."

Given this description one could write a thesis on the possible causes of Tjader's terminal event. One other early account contributed his death to the lingering effects of his arrow wounds sustained at Pyramid Lake. This is unlikely and his illness was probably due to heart or kidney failure. Dropsy is edema (swelling due to fluid retention) from heart or kidney disease. These diseases classically cause edema of the lower abdomen and legs, which is described in the above newspaper article. In addition, congestive heart failure also causes fluid to accumulate in the lungs. The question is: what is the underlying disease process? If the heart is the primary organ, the possibilities include valvular and heart muscle disease (myocarditis). A coronary artery event is possible but unlikely in an individual of Tjader's age. Rheumatic fever, less prevalent today due to the use of antibiotics, was epidemic in the nineteenth century and is a prime suspect. Most of the kidney diseases that would produce massive edema were not accurately diagnosed until the 20th-century and many still are not clearly understood, but a rapidly progressive nephritis can't be ruled out. Given what we know about diseases in 1870, Tjader probably died from 'heart disease.'

IRREGULAR PHYSICIAN
Dr. Simeon L. Lee

Anton P. Sohn MD

One hundred and twenty-five years after the Civil War, a cohesive medical profession in the sense we recognize today did not practice medicine. A percentage of the population depended upon unorthodox medical practitioners known as irregulars, which included botanical healers, homeopaths, water-cure proponents, religious healers, chiropractors, Indian doctors, charlatans and many more. Regular physicians or allopaths, on the other hand, were not uniformly trained and many had marginal skills. Such was the scene when Dr. Simeon L. Lee left Illinois in 1870 and settled in Nevada.

Simeon L. Lee was born in Vandalia, Illinois, on September 4, 1844, and in his early twenties became a lieutenant colonel in the 8th Illinois Infantry. After the War of Retribution, he went to Cincinnati, Ohio, and for two nonconsecutive years attended the

Physiomedical Institute, an irregular school of medicine. In his words this school was chosen because: "I was a lad, comparatively, when I matriculated in the school from which my father's family physician graduated. Of course, I. then thought it the only college. I have, I think, grown wiser since."

Physiomedical schools were an outgrowth of Thomsonism, which popularized botanical remedies similar to Native American medicine. These schools were established from 1839 to 1850 in Ohio, Georgia, Alabama, Tennessee, Virginia, Massachusetts, and New York. They were founded by Alva Curtis, a botanical healer, who split off from the Thomsonians.

As can be seen from Lee's statement, he tried to distance himself from irregular physicians, who practiced what is known as eclectic medicine. He appeared to be successful in this attempt, and was accepted by regular (allopathic) physicians. His advancement in professional status in Nevada is documented by his application and letter quoted above on letterhead from the Board of Registration and Examination to the U.S. Military requesting appointment as surgeon in the Nevada National Guard. He was the first president of the Nevada State Board of Health and at one time was secretary of the Board of Registration and Examination. According to his letter, he was voted into this position by his associates, of which all but one were 'regular' physicians.

After arriving in Nevada, Lee was 'in charge' of the Pioche, Lincoln County Hospital, Nevada National Guard from 1875 to 1879, 'in charge' of the Carson City Hospital from 1879 until at least 1901 (except 1893-4) and a railroad surgeon for the Virginia & Truckee and Carson & Colorado railroads for twenty years.

Military service was always a part of Dr. Lee's career. After his military service in Illinois, he was commissioned in 1877 as a major and inspector general in the Nevada National Guard and later advanced to the rank of colonel.

In a letter, he stated that he was the "only surgeon with Nevada National Guard in the war with Indians in what is known as the White Pine Indian War." Interestingly, no mention is made of the war in Nevada history books.

Dr. Lee also was an avid collector, and collected stamps, arrowheads, baskets, stones, ceramics, fossils, guns, and other rare objects. His widow presented his collection to the state of Nevada in 1934. This material became a cornerstone of the state collection in Carson City. As a result of military and community service and dedication to his adopted state Dr. Simeon Lee was an important Nevada physician and citizen until his death in 1927.

Vol. III, No. 3, Winter 1992-3

EDITORS NOTE:

Dr. Simeon Lee came to Pioche in 1872 and moved to Carson City in 1879. He is said to have been the first doctor to deliver an Indian baby. (Nevada State Historical Society records) The story is that Dr. Lee's help was asked, and the father was forcibly ejected from the Indian camp before the doctor could do the delivery. Dr. Lee also amputated an Indian's leg while he was practicing in Lincoln County. A picture is said to exist of the operation with someone holding the amputated leg.

Dr. Lee's microscope, which he brought to Pioche, is exhibited in the Arlene and Anton Sohn Museum at the School of Medicine and is probably the first microscope in Nevada. The silver nameplate from his office is also under his picture in the library.

Some information in this article was obtained from the "Simeon L. Lee Papers," National Library of Medicine, Bethesda, Maryland. Thanks also to Eileen Barker who obtained material about Dr. Lee from the Nevada State Museum and the Nevada Historical Society.

DR. SELDEN A. MCMEANS

Selden Allen McMeans was an important civic-minded doctor who was present at the birth of Nevada, but he was also a rabble-rouser for the South during the War Between the States. He was born in July 1806 near Knoxville, Tennessee, and later moved to Greenville, South Carolina, where he began his career in medicine.

When the war with Mexico began in 1846, Dr. McMeans left his plantation to volunteer for military service. In July 1849 he was in Mexico City, but he was planning to move to California. He ultimately settled in Sacramento, where he jumped into politics.

The Democratic State Convention elected McMeans one of twelve vice-presidents in 1852, and on January 1, 1854, he was installed as treasurer of the newly formed State of California, a post he held for two years. In November 1855 the State Council of the American Party in California, which supported the South's position on slavery, elected Dr. McMeans president.

In the fall of 1859 the cry for secession from the Union was growing, but the cry for Silver in the Nevada Territory was louder, and McMeans moved to Virginia City. There, he and a friend from California, Judge David Terry, organized support for the Confederacy by forming the Knights of the Golden Circle in John Newman's house, the first 'permanent' structure in Virginia City.

Besides being a politician and maybe a part-time miner, McMeans practiced medicine. Drs. McMeans and Edmund Gardner Bryant (cousin of poet William Cullen Bryant and married to Marie Louise, who later married mining mogul John Mackay) treated most of the miners in town for drinking water contaminated with 'arsenic,' etc. Julia Bulette, a well-known Virginia City prostitute, is also alleged to have cared for the miners, but there is no historical evidence to verify this.

On April 12, 1861, came news of the South firing on Fort Sumter, its surrender, and the secession of South Carolina. Tennessean McMeans sprang to action for the South and announced his plans to capture Fort Churchill and claim the territory for Jefferson Davis. The Confederate flag was raised over Newman's saloon, and Dr. McMeans organized 200 members of the Knights of the Golden Circle to defend the building. With the news of a detachment of soldiers from Fort Churchill being sent to Virginia City, Dr. McMeans and his supporters evaporated.

During the Civil War McMeans organized the Democratic Party in Nevada and was its first chairman. After the war, Dr. McMeans continued his political activities, and on June 22, 1872 he organized the Pacific Coast Pioneers at Virginia City. To be eligible one had to be male or a direct male descendent of a resident in one of the Pacific Coast States on January 1, 1851. The society acquired a building and had 400 members. Dr. Elias B. Harris who is discussed in this edition of *Greasewood*, was president of the society in 1881. Dr. Sheldon McMeans eventually relocated his practice in Reno. He died at the age of 70 in his Reno office July 31, 1876.

EDITORS' NOTE:

References: Sonoma County Historical Society's "The McMeans Family" by Connor, *The Saga of the Comstock Lode* by Lyman, and Thompson and West's *History of Nevada*.

Vol. XV, No. 1, Spring 2004

DOCTOR IN THE CIVIL WAR
DR. ELIAS HARRIS

Elias Braman Harris was born September 23, 1827, in Otsego County, New York. He attended Fairfield Academy and Geneva College where he studied medicine under Professor Frank Hamilton. In 1845 he enrolled in the two-year course in medicine at New York Medical University, one of the top medical schools in the country. After practicing in New York for two years, he eventually made his way to California by way of Panama and arrived in San Francisco in 1850.

He settled briefly in Calaveras County, which is now known for its vineyards and Mark Twain's humorous story about jumping frogs. Disgusted with frontier justice and witnessing a lynching, he stayed only a few months before moving to Ione in Amador Co.

There, he became involved in politics, opened a hotel, and leased a mine, the Oneida Mill and Mine. Dr. Harris is credited with building the first Nevada Territory steam quartz mill in 1860.

When the Civil War broke out, he returned east and joined the Union Army as a surgeon with the rank of major. After the war he married and returned to Virginia City where he practiced from 1875 until 1881. He also had a practice in Sacramento. Harris died in San Francisco, California, August 7, 1900.

Vol. XV, No. 1, Spring 2004

DOCTOR AND HIS STREET
Dr. George Thoma

Owen C. Bolstad MD

Dr. George H. Thoma may have been one of the most widely known and highly respected physicians who practiced medicine in Nevada during the second half of the 19th-century. His importance merited a street in Reno named in his honor. Today, Thoma Street is located two blocks north of the Veterans Administration Medical Center in Reno and runs from Virginia Street to Yori.

George was born on October 14, 1843, in Montgomery County, New York. His father was an emigrant from Germany who made his living as a clock maker. His mother was also born in Montgomery and was of Dutch descent. George received his primary education in Amsterdam, New York, then he enrolled at Albany Medical College where he earned his MD degree in 1864.

Immediately after graduation from Albany, Dr. Thoma volunteered for the Union Army and was designated as an assistant surgeon with the Second New York Artillery Regiment. He served with the Army of the Potomac until the surrender of the Confederate Army at Appomattox, where he was present to observe the flag of truce that signaled the end of the Civil War.

About one year after the cessation of hostilities, attracted by the reports of mineral wealth and driven by a spirit of adventure, Dr. Thoma set out for the western frontier. By the time he reached the Missouri River, he had spent his meager savings and was forced to sign on with a freighting outfit in order to continue his journey. After reaching Salt Lake City, he resigned his job with the freight company and set out walking across the Great Salt Desert with two companions and a mule pulling their supplies on a small cart. They arrived at the Reese River Valley during the summer of 1867 more dead than alive.

At first he took employment as an ore sorter in a stamp mill in an effort to finance his immediate needs. By 1868, he began practicing his profession of medicine once again in the Austin area. Sometime later he moved his practice to Eureka, where he maintained a successful practice for fourteen years. George Thoma immersed himself in his medical practice and into the affairs of his community as well. It has been said that he would answer a call to a miner's hut as readily as he would to the home of a wealthy man. He was well respected and in 1884, he was elected to the Nevada Senate where he served for four years.

In 1887, Dr. Thoma moved his practice to Reno, where he practiced until his death January 30, 1907, at the age of sixty-four. He was well thought of by his colleagues.

George Thoma loved his adopted state and often spoke of the peace he felt as he viewed Nevada's rugged mountains He lived and worked in Nevada for 40 years and during that time he contributed a great deal to that young and growing western state.

EDITORS' NOTE:

Reference: March 1907 *California State Journal of Medicine*. Mr. Albert R. Paulson of Menlo Park, California, brought it to our attention.

Vol. V, No. 2, Summer 1994

EXTRAORDINARY DOCTORS
Dawson, Bergstein, Thoma, and Lewis

Ryan Davis, History Student

Alson Dawson, Henry Bergstein, George Thoma, and John Lewis were extraordinary doctors, who are lost in time because they practiced one hundred years ago. In the following article, we will describe the importance of these four doctors, not only to the development of surgery in Nevada, but as leaders in medicine in the 19th-century.

On March 22, 1888, these four men set the standard in Nevada for medical advancement by performing a surgical procedure, which had never been attempted in this state. This procedure, known in the medical profession as an ovarian serous/mucinous cystadenectomy, was regarded as a dangerous operation. The first doctor in America to perform removal of this kind of an ovarian tumor was Ephraim McDowell (1771-1830). He operated on a kitchen table in Kentucky in 1809.

Many physicians in Nevada condemned the operation in 1888 that was performed by Dr. Alson Dawson and assisted by Thoma, Bergstein, and Lewis, as a disastrous venture. They believed the state simply did not have the adequate medical facilities or people with adequate training to master such a daunting challenge. In both McDowell's and the present case, the tumor was so large that pregnancy was considered. Furthermore, if the tumor was malignant or the contents of the benign cyst spilled in the abdomen, it could seed throughout the intestines and cause bowel obstruction and death.

The patient who became the first Nevadan to undergo the procedure was fifty-year-old Louise Ancker, who resided in Washoe City. Dr. Dawson diagnosed the plight of Mrs. Ancker four months prior to surgery. He thought the cyst was benign, but by its mere size threatened the healthy function of other internal organs. Mrs. Ancker was informed of the procedure's dangers and elected to have the operation done despite its risks.

The surgery was accomplished in one and a half hours in the old two-story Washoe Hospital building at Kirman and Mill Streets.

Done with great precision and delicacy was the main reason for its success.

Careful preparation went into the endeavor. Most of the instruments used were sterilized using a carbolized spray, and every nurse involved in the operation was required to take an antiseptic bath. Though routine as it may appear to many physicians today, these preparation techniques were all new and key to the procedure's success.

Many of these men accomplished more in the field of medicine than most doctors could hope to accomplish in a lifetime. Dr. Alson Dawson, besides being a prominent physician for over twenty years, was also one of the founders of the Nevada State Mental Hospital (nsmh), and was its first superintendent. Though no longer referred to by this name, the institution is still in service today as the Northern Nevada Adult Mental Health Services on Galetti Way in Sparks. Dawson, born in New York in 1844, left no record of where he received his MD. He was removed from his position as nsmh superintendent for an unknown reason shortly after the start of 1883. He died at the age of fifty-one from injuries sustained when his horse lost control on September 15, 1895, in Reno.

Each of Bergstein's assisting physicians served as superintendent of nsmh as well, and was a founding member of the first medical staff at Saint Mary's Hospital. Dr. Henry Bergstein, in addition to serving in the Nevada Legislature in 1875, was the father of the Nevada Medical Law of 1875, which required all doctors to present a medical license to the county recorder before they could practice in Nevada. Bergstein was one of seven members who formed the first organized medical society in Nevada in 1897. He attended Cooper Medical College (now Stanford Medical School) in 1872, and again in 1905. He died in San Francisco in 1918.

Dr. John Lewis served as president of nsma in 1909. He also served on the Nevada Board of Medical Examiners and was a member of the ama until his death in 1924.

Dr. George Thoma came to Nevada from New York after being an assistant surgeon in the Union Army. After settling in Eureka, Nevada, in 1867, he served in the Nevada Senate before moving to Reno to practice in 1887. Before his death in Reno in 1907, he served as president of nsma.

Pioneers and trailblazers in the field of medicine, these men proved that Nevada had the resources to accomplish what many believed was impossible. They formed the basis of Nevada's healthcare.

Vol. XIV, No. 2, Summer 2003

1867 SURGERY, DR. C.C. GREEN

Richard Pugh, former nsma ceo

Alfred Doten:

February 11, 1867, 1 went with Dr. C.C. Green (Virginia City 1864-1877) and helped him to perform an operation on the head of Mr. C.R. Gates—Near Summit Mill—He was hit with a stone playfully thrown at him at American Flat some 8 months ago—has hurt him ever since—Dr. now raised his scalp just over the left temple and took out several small pieces of bone and some granulations that had formed, sewed up wound, and put him to bed—He stood it like a major, taking no chloroform—suffered much pain however—Dr. gave me $5.00 for assisting him. I put item in the paper about it.

EDITORS' NOTE:

Reference: *The Journals of Alfred Doten 1849-1903*, edited by Walter Van Tilburg Clark, University of Nevada. Dr. C.C. Green was born in Ohio, but little is known about him.

Vol. I, No. 2, Spring 1990

BLACK DOCTOR ON THE COMSTOCK
Dr. W.H.C. Stephenson

Elmer R. Rusco PhD

Nevada's small black population during the 19th-century included a physician who practiced on the Comstock for at least twelve years. Dr. W.H.C. Stephenson was also an outstanding and respected leader of his African American community and also of the wider community of the preeminent mining and population center during this critical period in Nevada's early history. In addition to his medical contributions, he led the racial discrimination protest.

We do not know where Dr. Stephenson received his training, although apparently he was from Rhode Island. In 1867. he wrote, "I am a practicing physician and have my diploma and passed a successful examination before entering upon the practice of medicine." In 1868, he wrote that he had been practicing medicine for twenty years; if this is correct he must have become a physician around 1848, when he would have been twenty-three years-old.

We know that he was living in Sacramento and Marysville in 1862 or 1863. He first appears in a Comstock directory in 1863, where his address was given as a laundry on South G Street between Smith and Washington. The same directory lists him as a trustee and clerk of the First Baptist (Colored) Church, which was organized April 26, 1863. This was the first Baptist church on the Comstock.

Dr. Stephenson practiced medicine on the Comstock, mostly in Virginia City, Gold Hill, Silver City, and Dayton; in addition he took trips back east. Various sources list his office in Virginia City, usually on C Street, in 1864-1865, 1867, 1868-1869, 1871-1872, and 1875. In an 1878-'79 directory his wife was listed as living at the 120 South C Street address, which he had used for an office.

In several advertisements Dr. Stephenson described himself as an "eclectic physician." Eclectics had their own medical schools and a National Eclectic Medical Society before the Civil War.

Besides the obvious factor of favoring treatment procedures from a variety (hence, eclectic) of different sources, eclectic physicians at this time were noted for their avoidance of a wide variety of harsh medicines or methods of treatment—such as purgation, lancing, the promotion of fevers, and the prescription of mercury compounds—which were then not uncommon among physicians. In these respects eclectics often provided better—because less harmful—care than many other physicians of the day.

The statements made by him about a diploma and passage of some kind of examination suggests the Dr. Stephenson graduated from an eclectic medical school, but further research is needed. As the editor has pointed out, "Not all those who called themselves physicians were educated in the healing arts. Licensing laws were virtually non-existent and educational requirements had not yet been established to ensure that all physicians were trained."

In 1868, the Comstock's pioneer black physician wrote a column on smallpox, which was printed in the *Territorial Enterprise*. In it he reported that this disease had been spreading in San Francisco and several other California cities, had reached Gold Hill and Virginia City, and had become a matter about which Nevada citizens ought to be alarmed. He offered several suggestions for "prevention and mitigation" of smallpox on the Comstock, starting with vaccination but including "total abstinence from all intoxicating liquors," the "destruction of all bedding used by persons who have been afflicted with the disease" and disinfecting houses where there had been patients ill with the disease. Dr. Stephenson ended by advising physicians to change their clothing after treating smallpox patients. He offered the opinion that not all physicians would do this and, "To this negligence of the medical profession in San Francisco is due, in part, the present increase of the smallpox."

Nevada's first black physician was obviously well educated and quite intelligent, as a number of letters to the editor and his leadership in various community matters attest. In 1870, when black men were allowed to vote for the first time after the 15th Amendment.

Dr. Stephenson and other black Nevadans registered to vote. The *Territorial Enterprise* reported, "A person of lighter skin but darker heart refused to register because he would not place his name under the Doctor's." The newspaper offered the opinion that Stephenson would not have objected to placing his name after that of this man because, "Dr. Stephenson has intelligence enough to see that it would not detract from him to have his name follow that of an inferior."

His important role in the first Baptist church on the Comstock has been noted. The "first pastor of this church, Rev. Charles Satchel left after about a year and was succeeded as minister by Dr. Stephenson. However, the church ran into debt and the building was sold at auction in 1866. Some members of the congregation criticized Dr. Stephenson when he purchased the building and kept the proceeds.

When Nevada became a separate territory in 1861 and a state in 1864, there were various "relics" "of the barbarism of slavery imprinted in the statute books of Nevada, as an 1865 address to Nevada citizens from a black organization headed by Dr. Stephenson put it. For example, the suffrage was restricted to white males, "Negroes, Mongolians, and Indians" could not be educated in the public schools unless a separate school was set up for them.

Members of the same groups could not marry whites and these three groups were forbidden to testify against white persons in either civil or criminal cases (with the curious exception that Chinese were allowed to testify against whites). In the latter case, Dr. Stephenson was specifically affected to a substantial extent. In 1867 he protested: "… $3,000 due to me, in the State from Anglo-Saxons, for professional services, which I can only collect through sufferance; and this, in sums of 10 to $40, is a deal loss, from the fact that the parties have shielded themselves through an Art of the State which leaves me no redress."

In supporting his call for repeal of the testimony law in civil cases, the *Territorial Enterprise* asserted that Dr. Stephenson no doubt paid "more tax than both of the two legislators who had killed the bill to repeal this law during the 1867 session." Dr. Stephenson asserted in 1870, "My Country and State taxes for the year 1869, in gold coin, were $40, City tax $16, Government (federal occupational) tax $50."

Dr. Stephenson was one of the leaders of the African American community who protested these discriminatory laws and sought their repeal. During the 1865 legislative session, a petition requesting that African Americans be allowed to testify against whites in criminal cases was sent to the legislature and a bill allowing this, although ambiguously worded, was adopted. Dr. Stephenson, organized to end exclusion from voting, testimony, and the schools.

In a vigorous attack on the school law in 1870, the physician reported the taxes that he had paid during 1869 and protested that the exclusion of black taxpayers from the public schools was grossly unfair and a violation of the "right to an equal protection of the laws … and equal school rights with the Anglo-Saxon." He suggested that the question was whether "people of color" were "as human beings, entitled to any school privileges whatever." The 1870 census of population reported that Dr. Stephenson and his wife Jane had a daughter who was 13 in that year; no doubt his child was one of the children not allowed to attend public schools.

The efforts led by Dr. Stephenson were rebuffed in both the 1866 and 1867 legislative sessions and equal access to public schools was not achieved until 1872, when the Nevada Supreme Court declared the school law barring non-white children to be unconstitutional. The 1869 legislature repealed the law forbidding blacks to testify against whites in civil cases, while retaining it for other non-whites.

When black men secured the right to vote in 1870, a Lincoln Union Club was organized in Virginia City, "with Dr. Stephenson as president. This organization held an elaborate celebration of the passage of the 15th amendment on February 3, 1870, including a parade and a reading of the 1866 federal Civil Rights Act. While he did not give the main address at this event, Dr. Stephenson made a few remarks, which a newspaper called sensible and appropriate.

African American leaders after the Civil War were strongly Republican, because nationally this party had secured enactment of the 13th, 14th, and 15th amendments and several civil rights laws. When a Liberal Republican party was organized in 1872 and put forward Horace Greeley as its presidential candidate, Dr. Stephenson, even though he was at the time in New Rochelle, New York wrote a vigorous statement addressed to "Colored Voters of Storey County and Nevada." This document asserted that the Liberal Republicans and the Democrats were involved in "a league against Emancipation (and) against the Civil Rights bill" and the 14th and 15th amendments. He urged black voters in Nevada to vote for the reelection of President Grant and for the "old Republican party," which was still devoted to freedom and equal rights.

In short, W.H.C. Stephenson was not only a physician on the Comstock for a decade and a half but was also an early advocate of human rights in the state. He deserves to be remembered for these achievements.

EDITORS' NOTE:

Dr. Elmer R. Rusco is professor emeritus in political science at the UNR.

Vol. IX, No. 2, Summer 1998

WASHOE CITY'S NINE DOCTORS

Eileen Barker, UNSOM Pathology Department Manager

During the ten-year period 1861-1871, for varying periods of time, nine physicians practiced medicine in Washoe City, Nevada. Those physicians were Drs. L. Kords, T.C. Allen, B.B. Bonham, G.A. Weed, J.S. Stackpole, W.P.L. Winiham, A.P. Mitchell, Simeon Bishop, and Henry Hogan. A short history of the rise of Washoe City in November 1861 provides the *raison d'être* for so many physicians in the small city.

Farming and livestock production by the white man in Nevada began in the Carson Valley in the spring of 1851. Other settlers moved in and extended farming and ranching operations into Washoe Valley where the town of Franktown became settled in 1852. In the nearby mountains the discovery in 1859 of rich gold and silver deposits—the Comstock Lode of Virginia City—had an immediate effect on the small valley. The towns of Ophir, Little Bangor, Mill Station, Galena, and Washoe City soon blazed up. The little settlements took on an importance and growth that lasted for several years.

In 1861, Washoe City became the seat of justice for the County of Washoe, one of nine original counties of the Territory of Nevada. Washoe City's population of 543 tripled within the year. Saloon keepers, lawyers, businessmen, journalists, carpenters, masons, general laborers, school teachers, doctors and one dentist moved into the bustling town. By the mid-1860s the population of Washoe City and surrounding towns reached 6,000.

Washoe City had the first stock exchange in the West, prior to the San Francisco exchange.

The absence of food, water and lumber on the Comstock compelled Virginia City to look to the Washoe Valley to meet the needs of its burgeoning population. Lying between the Virginia Range and the Carson Range, the fertile valley was a natural meadow that provided the agriculture, while the nearby dense growth of pine and fir supplied the lumber. The one lumber mill in Franktown was soon operating to the limit of its capacity; within a short time there were fifteen sawmills in and around Washoe City, all in full operation.

Millwrights, lumberjacks, log wagon bullwhackers, teamsters, and machinists moved in. Great quantities of lath, shingles and lumber for buildings and large timber to shore up the many mine excavations were sent by freight wagons up the steep grade to the bustling Comstock Lode. Washoe Valley farmers shipped prodigious amounts of hay, alfalfa, barley, oats, vegetables, fruit, beef, poultry, butter, hops for beer production, and honey.

By all accounts these early settlers were a healthy bunch, but epidemics, accidents in the mills, shootings, fights and other trauma provided the demand for medical services. Doctors arrived, some to heal and, since those were days of gold-rush fever, some came because of their own 'fever.' The state law requiring presentation of a medical diploma to the county recorder was not enacted until 1875, so little is known of the educational backgrounds of these early physicians. Sam P. Davis in *History of Nevada* notes, "Of their ability in the profession no one knew and very few cared.

The doctors honored the community with their presence and the people, wishing to be sociable, gave them employment." It is known that Simeon Bishop was born in 1833 in Pennsylvania, and was educated at the Physiomedical Institute of Cincinnati. Henry Hogan, a native of Vermont, received his medical education at the Burlington Academy of Vermont Medical College. Dr. Mitchell was from New York, but nothing is known of his educational background. Dr. Kords lived in Galena, was an active member of the Union political party, practiced medicine as a profession, and operated a successful poultry business. Dr. Winiham ran the drugstore in Washoe City. Dr. G.A. Weed became Superintendent of Schools, Washoe Co. Nov. 3, 1863.

When an 1862 smallpox in the population around Watson's Mill continued unabated, the Washoe County Commissioners in the summer of 1864 purchased the Printing Office Building in Washoe City for $1,000 and converted it into a hospital. A tax of 20¢ on each $100 of property value was levied to cover the cost of caring for the sick. Dr. Weed was awarded a contract for $2.50 a day to treat, feed and supply medicine for the patients.

Meteoric as its rise, so too followed the end of the towns of the valley changes occurred and the economy of Washoe City collapsed. At the same time that the smelting and lumber mills were built in Washoe Valley, others were erected at Gold Hill, Seven-Mile

Canyon and along the Carson River. The Comstock's dependence on the mills of Washoe Valley lessened.

In 1869, the Virginia and Truckee Railroad was completed from Carson City to Virginia City, and the ore could be carried to the mills on the river much more cheaply than it could be hauled over the mountain by freight wagons, while wood and lumber could be shipped by rail from those mills closer to the Comstock. The milling business in Washoe City rapidly died and the town's twin mainstays were gone. With the transcontinental completion of the Central Pacific Railroad in May 1869, the city of Reno became the hub of commerce. The final death knell tolled for Washoe City in 1879-'81 when Reno was named the county seat of Washoe County, and all county business was moved out of Washoe City.

In the manner of the tumbleweeds rolling over the valley, some of the physicians who lived and practiced in Washoe City passed through the area leaving scant trace of their presence there or their activities after leaving. Of others, more information is found. Dr. Henry Hogan became the Washoe County Physician in 1874. Dr. Hogan was active in the Populist Party and became a state assemblyman in 1898. He died of pneumonia March 17, 1902, in Reno, Nevada. Dr. Simeon Bishop moved to Reno, and in 1884 became the superintendent of the Nevada State Hospital. He died in San Francisco, California, on February 8, 1920, of generalized arteriosclerosis. Of interest to Nevada history buffs is the fact that Dr. Bishop's daughter was married to Comstock's *Territorial Enterprise* noted editor, Wells Drury. In 1936 Drury authored the book *An Editor on the Comstock Lode*, his reminiscences of Comstock society after his arrival in the early 1870s.

EDITORS' NOTE:

The settlements of Ophir and Galena have long disappeared. Franktown has returned to its pastoral, bucolic setting. Today, in the middle of one of its meadows where cattle once grazed lies a new golf course surrounded by up-scale building sites. In Washoe City one crumbling commercial building is left standing. A well-preserved cemetery remains.

Vol. VI, No. 3, Autumn 1995

SCHOOL SUPERINTENDENT
DR. HAMIS S. HERRICK

During the fall of 1867 rich silver deposits were discovered near Hamilton, Nevada. At that time Hamilton was the county seat of White Pine County, and with the rapid influx of miners that city soon became a real boomtown. It was estimated that the population of Hamilton and the surrounding mining camps reached upwards of 30,000 people at the height of the mining activity. The mining bonanza soon played out, and the transient miners and their followers began to leave for other places. Within a period of twenty years, the once bustling city of Hamilton was fast becoming a ghost town, and after a disastrous fire burned down the Court House in Hamilton, the county seat was moved to Ely.

Dr. Hamis S. Herrick was a native of New York and had received his medical education at an eastern medical school. Dr. Herrick began the practice of medicine in California several years before he moved to Hamilton, Nevada, in 1869. For some undisclosed reason his wife and family had remained in the east when the doctor moved out west to seek his fortune.

During this long separation from his family he maintained communication with his family with a series of letters to his daughter. These letters, covering the period from 1881 to 1891 were preserved and are now available in the Nevada Historical Society in Reno. A study of these letters gives a look at the practice of medicine in rural Nevada during the late 1800s. Nothing in his letters indicates whether or not Dr. Herrick's family ever joined him in Nevada, or if he ever returned to his home in New York.

Dr. Herrick played an active role in his community, acting as county physician for many years and served a number of terms as County Superintendent of Schools.

He also owned and operated a drug store, where in addition to drugs and medicines he sold groceries and other sundry items.

In a transcript of the letters to his daughter published by Russell R. Elliott in a "*Nevada Historical Society Quarterly*," are these references to Dr. Herrick's medical practice: "...You speak about smallpox. I was vaccinated when a child and then about twenty years ago, have been a great deal exposed since, but have never taken it although it does not hurt to be vaccinated once in ten years. It has been terrible in Troy (New York) during the past winter hundreds have died. It has been very bad in San Francisco and also in Virginia City (Nevada). It has not been here since 1869. I have attended persons in all diseases in which flesh is heir to but of all loathsome, which caps the climax, I must say smallpox takes the preference."

Dr. Herrick had suffered a paralytic stroke some time in 1881, and reports on his own health" "I feel very much better to think I am again able to be around and see to my affairs. I can't write yet with that facility I could before I was taken sick, still I am gradually gaining under numerous tonics. I was not out Christmas or New Years to take any dinners, lots of eatables were brought to me. I have many good-hearted friends in these regions. Everybody called when I was sick. I did not want for anything, did not have any expense except watchers. It cost $8 per day, for men to be on hand. It is very expensive to be sick here, at the best. Still it don't trouble me if I only fully recuperate.

After a vacation trip to California he writes: "I ought to have remained longer in California, but was obliged to come back on account of more patients in the hospital. The Doctor I left in charge did not give satisfaction, consequently.

I was obliged to return or resign which I did not want to do as long as I do business in Hamilton... We have to ride in wagons forty-five miles over hills and mountains before arriving at the narrow gage railroad, then go ninety miles when we are at the Central Pacific then 600 miles to San Francisco. It costs heavily to travel in this country. My passage down and back was $108."

While at the Bay City I took Turkish baths every other day, it wouldn't do to take them every day. They are too weakening. The first operation is to sit in an easy chair in a hot room till the perspiration flows freely. Then go into another room and perspire still more freely than in the first. This takes an hour or more, and then a man goes through manipulations with water and soap by rubbing and brushing. Then one is put under a shower bath of tepid water after which another rubbing is over, then one is wrapped in woolen blankets and sleep as long as you please, on rising another shower bath is given and rubbing, then dress and sit in a comfortable room and read papers ½ hour, this ends the program.

In June 1883, he writes: "...I have had more mountain fever than any spring since I came to Hamilton. Some days I have had as high as eight or ten patients with mountain fever, which is a nervous, low-type of bilious fever. If a physician understands it is easily treated. The fever lasts from twelve to twenty-four hours under proper treatment and while under it they generally think they are going to die. Women, if on the order of hysterical are to die, but I have never lost any by this complaint. A number of New York gentlemen and ladies are out here at present. All have had the fever and I have brought all of them safely through. They are very "tony." The first one taken sick was the President of the Company. I was sent for, he began by giving his orders. Interrogated by asking him if he or I was the physician, he said that was his custom in N.Y. I deliberately informed him that it was not according to my practice. He said that he did not want my attendance. Left, about fifteen hours afterward I was sent for."

"He had got a quack, who has three or four things to give, this N.Y. gent begged me with his wife and daughters to take hold of his case and in two hours the fever began to go down from 100 degrees to 98 degrees. It took a week to get him around as he is a man hard on seventy years.

Dr. Herrick died from a stroke in 1891 without ever returning to his home in the East.

EDITORS' NOTE:

References: "Letters From A Nevada Doctor to His Daughter In Connecticut, 1881-1891" and found in the *Nevada Historical Society Quarterly*, Volumes 1, 2, and 3, summer and fall of 1957. Information is from Lee Mortensen.

Vol. IV, No. 1, Spring 1993

UNIVERSITY OF NEVADA'S FIRST SCHOLARSHIP
Dr. W. H. Patterson

Dr. William H. Patterson, played many roles during his lifetime as a soldier, a husband, a father, a rancher, a horseman, a physician, a statesman, and an administrator. He fought for and represented his country, saved lives and lost a few, made fortunes and lost fortunes, enjoyed good health and suffered from blindness. He experienced much love and suffered much loss.

He was a risk-taker as described by Dr. Frank Farwell, a consulting psychologist to the U.S. Congress, who developed a theory that the U.S. population is largely a nation of risk-takers "made up of the descendants of immigrants who took the supreme risk of uprooting themselves to come to the New World—thrill seekers who need a higher degree of stimulation than others to be fulfilled."

Both Dr. Patterson's parents had separately immigrated to Canada in the 1830s, to seek a better life. His mother, Elizabeth Smith was 212

born in Johnston, Renreshire, Scotland, in 1817 and arrived in Canada in 1836. Soon after her arrival she met John Patterson, also a Scottish immigrant and they were married in 1839.

They had five children, including William H. Patterson, who was born in 1843.

The family settled in Almonte, Ontario, Canada, in a stable and secure environment. Elizabeth was widely known for her good works and kindness in the community. Her obituary in the local newspaper spoke of "her quiet and unassuming manner and Christian integrity that won the admiration of all with whom she came in contact." Upward mobility appeared to thrive in the Patterson children, both William and his brother James graduated from McGill's Medical School, sister Jessie became head of the art department at the university, brother Robert became chief of the Canadian Supreme Court, and sister Mary married a businessman.

Most of his siblings made a good life for themselves, never living far from the family home in Almonte, but William H. Patterson had the *wanderlust*. Soon after his graduation from McGill University with honors he made plans to leave for the United States. The reason for his departure is unknown. Eastern Canada was peaceful at that time, there was no family discord, and his future seemed assured. William was a risk-taker, and the appeal of the Wild West may have stirred his adventurous spirit—at any rate he moved to Arizona in 1867 and applied for United States citizenship.

He spent four years as an assistant surgeon in Arizona with the United States Army, then, he moved to San Francisco. With a new contract with the U.S. Army, he served at Fort Bidwell, Modoc County in Northern California as assistant surgeon from March 20, 1872, until October 1, 1873. In this time period, Dr. Patterson served in the Lava Beds during the Modoc Indian Wars made famous by the Indian warrior Captain Jack.

When his military career ended, he set up medical practice near Fort Bidwell in Cedarville, Modoc County, California. There he married the town's schoolteacher, Mary Drouillard, in 1874.

Miss Drouillard graduated from one of the first classes at San Jose Teacher's College, which later became San Jose State University. They had four children. His medical practice built up rapidly and Dr. Patterson was most welcomed in the community. According to the local newspaper: "There was no doctor nearer on the south than Reno, on the west than Susanville, and the east than Omaha, and on the north there was nobody at all."

He set all the broken bones, cured all the fevers, and brought in all the babies in Modoc County, California, Roop County, Nevada, and Lake and Grant Counties in Oregon. He covered an area at least 150 square miles. To cover these long distances he kept a number of fine saddle horses, and on a long ride he would change horses once or twice, leaving his horse on the road and hiring a person to ride out and back. It was said that he had the largest surgical practice in the United States.

As a successful businessman he began to buy land. He bought the Cottonwood Ranch in Surprise Valley, near Cedarville. He bought the Duck Lake Ranch in addition to their home in Cedarville He invested in property near Tonopah, Nevada. Patterson Lake in Surprise Valley was named after him.

He was a member of Surprise Valley Lodge No. 235, Free and Accepted Masons and served as Worthy Master of that Lodge. He was elected as California State Senator representing Modoc, Lassen, Sierra, and Plumas Counties from 1887 to 1888. While in the senate he introduced numerous bills involving Napa State Hospital, Chinese immigrants, and the mining industry.

In 1899, he accepted an appointment from Governor Sadler of Nevada to serve as Superintendent of the Nevada State Hospital, so he moved his family to Sparks, Nevada. Two years later in 1902, wife Mary died at the age of forty-six years. Dr. Patterson established the first scholarship at the University of Nevada with a gift of $100. He later married schoolteacher from Cedarville, Annie Stevens. Within about ten years he separated from his wife and moved back to Cedarville.

Like many professional men in that time, Dr. Patterson invested in gold mining operations, and apparently made a great deal of money. However, his last investment in the Hess Gold Mining and Milling Company was not successful, and he lost a lot of money.

In his retirement Dr. Patterson was an avid reader with a love of poetry. He is remembered as a real gentleman, impeccably dressed, with an erect posture. He insisted upon proper English and disliked nicknames. In the later years of his life he lost his vision. No longer able to care for himself, he moved in with one of his daughters in

Berkeley, California. On March 29, 1925, he died in the Alta Bates Hospital in Berkeley at the age of 82.

EDITORS' NOTE:

Reference: Biography by Dr. William H. Patterson's granddaughter, Mrs. Beatrice Rey. Granddaughter Mabel P. Baker and great granddaughter Margaret Key Duensing furnished additional information and pictures.

Vol. X, No. 3, Fall 1999

ALMOST FORGOTTEN PHYSICIAN
DR. SAMUEL W. WEAVER

Richard A. Sumin

Greasewood Press' *The Healers of 19th-Century Nevada* published the names of over 700 doctors who have practiced in the territory or State of Nevada between 1857 and 1900. Obviously this list is not complete because in the early days, for various reasons, doctors came to the state, stayed a short time, and left no records. Prior to 1899 when the Nevada Legislature created the Nevada Board of Medical Examiners, some county records were incomplete and even destroyed. Furthermore, only names and dates of some doctors survived. Others left only their name. Therefore, when we are alerted to a new name or more information about an individual, we want to record the information for our history of medicine archives, and alert our readers who might have more information.

In 1999, we received a letter from Richard A. Sumin of Battle Mountain, a relative of Dr. Samuel W. Weaver, who practiced in Paradise Valley. Mr. Sumin sent us a history and photograph of Dr. Weaver from the *1912 Centennial History of Oregon*. He also noted the Weaver's arrival was announced in the *Silver State*, a Humboldt County newspaper on April 25, 1884.

Samuel Weaver was born in Canonsburg. Pennsylvania, on January 9, 1853. He attended a local academy before graduating from the College of Physicians and Surgeons in Baltimore in 1882. After two years of practice in his home state, the young bachelor moved to Paradise Valley, Nevada, in 1884 where he remained for two years. No information is recorded as to why he left Nevada. Maybe the mines played out, maybe there were no eligible young women, or maybe he moved on for better economic opportunities. At any rate he settled in Hubbard, Oregon, where he married and spent the rest of his life. In that community, he served on the city council and played first violin in the Hubbard Symphony Orchestra. According to the *Journal of the American Medical Association*, he died of heart disease October 10, 1924.

Vol. XIII, No. 2, Autumn 2002

TALE OF THE PHANTOM HAND
DR. JOHN D. CAMPBELL

Kimberly Campbell

Dr. J.D. Campbell of Pioche, Nevada, could have easily been the role model for Doc Baker of 'Little House on the Prairie,' or the famous 'Doc of Gun Smoke.' Like the role they portray, Dr. Campbell was a real life country doctor. Traveling by horse and wagon, regardless of weather conditions, to minister to humble homes or miner's cabin, Dr. John Dalgleish Campbell gave many years of professional care to the residents of Lincoln County.

Born in Hartland, Michigan, on July 9, 1853, Campbell graduated with honors from the University of Michigan Medical School. While in Michigan, he married Bertha Haford and fathered one son, Wilkes James Campbell. After the death of his wife Dr. Campbell moved west. He spent some time in White Pine County where he practiced medicine. He married Maggie Leahigh and soon after moved to Pioche. While in Pioche, they had three more children–two sons, Ainslie and Floyd, and a daughter Edith. The early death of Edith was a family tragedy.

In 1902, Dr. Campbell operated upon an Indian lady with cancer of the breast. During the operation he inadvertently cut himself and soon developed blood poisoning. Critically ill, he was taken to Delamore, Nevada, where there were two brothers practicing medicine. In a desperate attempt to save Dr. Campbell's life they amputated his left arm just above the elbow. He remained very ill for a long time, but eventually recovered. During his convalescence he began to suffer a lot of pain in his amputated hand, which had been buried in Delamore. He said that it felt like the fingers of his left hand were clenched together and cramping. The 'phantom pain' caused by neuromata growing in the stump of the amputated limb became almost unbearable. Finally his oldest son, Maggie Leahigh Wilkes James Campbell drove to Delamore by horse and wagon. He dug up the buried hand and straightened out the fingers. Almost simultaneously Dr. Campbell's pain ceased, and he was much relieved. His wife, Maggie, became his new left hand, assisting in bandaging and other treatments.

During the great influenza epidemic of 1917-18, Dr. Campbell and his son Wilkes would travel from house to house with a bucket of soup, giving soup to the ill and quarantined victims of the epidemic. He developed a reputation as 'guardian of the sick'..

On many a cold winter night the good doctor answered calls for assistance all across the county. With him and his son, Wilkes, bundled up in heavy bearskin coats and hats, they would drive many miles in a wagon or cutter.

Before they left on a call they would heat up rocks to help keep their feet warm, but that didn't do very much good as the rocks soon cooled. The cold was sometimes nearly unbearable, but Dr. Campbell never refused a call for help.

In addition to his medical practice, the good doctor was very active in community affairs. He was elected assemblyman from White Pine County in 1889, and beginning in 1906, he served two terms as a state senator. He presided over the Nevada Senate for one full session in the absence of the Lieutenant Governor. He was a 32nd degree Mason, an Elk, and an Odd fellow.

Dr. J.D. Campbell died at his home in Pioche on January 8, 1928, at the age of seventy-five years, much appreciated and respected as the 'Country Doctor' of Lincoln County.

EDITORS' NOTE:

Kimberly Campbell, great granddaughter of Dr. Campbell, submitted material for this story. Linwood W. Campbell, grandson of Dr. J.D. Campbell in 1998, took the information from a tape recording. We appreciate this contribution to the Medical History of Nevada. Linwood W. Campbell submitted portrait to the Great Basin History of Medicine collection.

Vol. X, No. 4, Winter 1999-2000

WOMEN PHYSICIANS
IN 19TH-CENTURY NEVADA

Anton P. Sohn MD

The typical medical practitioner in 19th-century Nevada was a white Euro-American male. After 1870 when the first woman noted to be a physician in Nevada, Helena Jones, practiced in Treasure City, White Pine County, women made progress in the profession. Doctress Hoffman, a woman medical practitioner and midwife, was listed in the Virginia City by the *Territorial Enterprise* in 1865, and by the end of the century, twenty-two women doctors were listed in Nevada.

Although the medical profession would continue to be dominated by men into the 20th-century, a steady expansion of the role of women in medicine was occurring.

By the mid-19th century, it became obvious that there was a need for women in medical practice. The 'Victorian' ideas of decency and modesty were a barrier to men who wished to practice gynecology and obstetrics. Although there were a few male physicians in the early 19th century who practiced midwifery, many women patients avoided them. Later, in some communities in the West, traditional Chinese doctors were more acceptable to women with 'female' problems than American trained physicians who were thought to be less sensitive to the needs of women.

Elizabeth Blackwell, the first woman graduate of an American medical school in 1848, was stimulated to study medicine when she observed the sufferings of a friend with a gynecological problem who had been seeing a male physician. However, the medical profession was divided on the education of women who wished to study medicine. Some felt that a male student should not study anatomy next to a female student and that women should study in all-female classes

For this reason in 1848, Samuel Gregory founded the New England Female Medical Education Society, which became the New England Female Medical College. His intent was not to create a medical college equal to existing male institutions, but to concentrate on graduating women who would be midwives. He termed his graduates 'Doctresses.' The term doctress dates back at least to 1800 when a doctress practiced medicine in Bethel, Maine. Gregory stressed that doctresses should be subservient to male doctors, charge less, and treat only the less difficult cases.

The first woman physician in Nevada who is verified to have graduated from a traditional medical college was Kate Nicholas Post. She graduated in 1879 from Cooper Medical College in San Francisco and practiced in Virginia City, Nevada in 1879.

Cooper and Toland Medical College (later, the University of California) were exemplary in graduating women physicians. Cooper graduated the first woman in 1877, and Toland graduated its first in 1878. From then until 1900, ten percent of Toland's graduates and 13.4 percent of Cooper's were women. Records show that at least twenty-two women had practiced medicine in Nevada prior to 1900, and about half of them graduated from allopathic medical schools. The twenty-two women comprise 3.4 percent of the physicians in Nevada before 1900. Statistics from the U.S. at the start of the twentieth century reveal that women comprised 5.0 percent of the physician population. These statistics are not completely comparable since one encompasses forty-nine years and the other represents one point in time, but they do demonstrate the small number of women practicing medicine in Nevada.

Vol. VI, No. 2, Summer 1995

EDITORS NOTE:

Kate Nicholas Post was born in Marshall, Illinois, in 1853 and graduated from Cooper Medical College in San Francisco in 1879. Shortly after graduation she moved to Virginia City, but by 1881 she was living on Mission Street in San Francisco. In 1883 she was practicing medicine at the Pacific Dispensary Hospital in San Francisco, and later that year on September 15 she married Dr. Leander Van Orden. By 1890 she was practicing at the Alameda Unitarian Clinic, and in 1930 she moved to Santa Cruz where she died June 9, 1953.

NEVADA WOMEN PHYSICIANS 1851-1900

Weed, Adaline	Washoe County, 1860-'67
Hoffman, 'Doctress'	Virginia City, 1865
Jones, 'Doctress' Helena	White Pine County, 1869
Buchins, 'Doctress'	Elko County, 1875
DeLong, C. E	Humboldt County, 1875

Anderson, Helen	Reno, 1875
Post, Kate	Virginia City, 1879
Seals, Ramlis	White Pine County, 1880
Clark, Elizabeth	White Pine County, 1880
Gray, Georgia	White Pine County, 1880
DeForest, Brown	Virginia City, 1880
Atwater, Hattie	Carson City, 1882
Newland, Ruth	Carson City, 1882
Sites, Ida	Lander County, 1888
Fee, Katherine	Washoe County, 1899
Geiss, Anna	Washoe County, 1889
Hastings, Carrie	Virginia City, 1892
Wilder, Annie	Virginia City, 1894
Longshore-Potts, 'Doctor'	Virginia City, 1897
Cook, Eliza	Douglas County, 1891
Albers, Annet	Washoe County, 1900
McGarver, Mary	Humboldt County, 1900

HOMEOPATHY ON THE COMSTOCK
DR. FREDERICK HILLER

Anita Watson, UNR Graduate Student

Medicine was unregulated in the state [and nation] during the 19th- century and anyone could practice medicine and be called a doctor. Furthermore, the cause of most disease was unknown and therefore homeopathy was a viable option for medical treatment. There were several successful physicians who practiced that philosophy during the 19th century in Nevada, but Dr. Frederick Hiller was prominent.

The philosophy of homeopathy embraces treatment with minute doses producing the same symptom as manifested by the disease process. Dr. Hiller was a successful homeopathic physician in Virginia City. The German physician Samuel Hahnemann devised homeopathy in the late 18th- century. He based his medical system on two laws, *similars similia similibus curantur* (use of a drug that produces the same symptoms as the disease) and *infintestinals* (the smaller the dose the more effective the treatment).

In actuality, drugs were diluted to the point where they had no effect.

This system appealed to many Americans who were fed up with harsh treatments–bloodletting, treatment with mercuric compounds to the point of poisoning, et cetera, by regular doctors. The homeopathic system spread rapidly across America and several medical schools expounding its philosophy were established. The most notable example was Hahnemann Medical College, which later became an allopathic medical school.

In Nevada, the conflict between homeopathic and allopathic physicians was waged most prominently on the Comstock. The well-known newspaperman, Alfred Doten, sided with homeopathy and Dr. Hiller. They published two pamphlets: "Common Sense vs. Allopathic Humbuggery" and "Medical Truths and Light for the Million."

Doten was hardly an unbiased, objective observer. He was paid by Hiller, assisted him in surgery, gave anesthesia during his operations, collected his medical bills, and defended him in the *Territorial Enterprise*. Doten pointed out that patients came to Hiller after treatment prescribed by allopathic doctors had failed.

In 1871, Dr. Hiller retired to San Francisco. In spite of the fact that allopathic doctors anathematized Hiller and homeopathic medicine, very few physicians at that time were homeopaths. Only five percent of practicing doctors in 19th-century Nevada had graduated from a homeopathic medical school. Obviously, with the lack of regulation or medical licensing in the state at that time, there could have been more physicians who had not graduated from a homeopathic medical school but adhered to its philosophy. However, it is unlikely that they constituted a significant number. Just the same, when conventional medicine cannot cure the patient or give him hope, alternative treatments are sought.

Vol. VI, No. 4, Winter 1995-'96

SURGEON FREDERICK HILLER

Richard G. Pugh, Former nsma ceo

Alfred Doten was a prolific recorder of life in Virginia City for over five decades. His diary not only captured the essence of a colorful era in early Nevada but also recorded helping doctors when they needed anesthesia for their patients. In his three-volume diary of 2,300 pages Doten recorded his daily activities, freelance writing for the *Territorial Enterprise*, "Assistance in medical procedures, and activities of hard rock miners." His canine companion, Keyzer, accompanied him in his travels and adventures during the frenetic gold-rush period.

Doten was particularly adept at painting a picture of the daily successes and excesses of flamboyant miners that resulted in violence necessitating a physician and anesthesia. He helped and frequently was called by local physicians to assist in surgical procedures by administering the preferred anesthesia chloroform. Records from Doten's diary indicate that he was one of the first 'lay anesthesiologists' in Nevada.

He recorded numerous gunfights in Virginia City and related the various ways in which disputes were settled. He wrote about a man who was struck with a miner's pick after a violent argument and nearly died. Virginia City justice was swift in that case as the assaulting man was summarily struck with the same pick for punishment.

Then, there was a case in 1864, where one of the townspeople was seriously injured, not in a gunfight or mine injury, but while exercising in a local gymnasium. Doten assisted Dr. Frederick Hiller in setting the patient's leg. On another occasion, Doten was called to assist the doctor in treating a man who was injured when his gun exploded while rabbit shooting. Two middle fingers were amputated while Doten administered the chloroform, and afterwards he wrote, "The gun was over-loaded and had not been shot for three weeks."

Doten later joined Dr. Heller in amputating the "preputium" (prepuce) of a miner living in the nearby community of Dutch Flats.

Infection of the foreskin was not uncommon in the 19th-century and was treated by circumcision. Life during the Comstock Lode era was often perilous never dull.

In addition to his medical duties, Doten participated in many of the 'cultural' activities of Virginia City such as performances at Piper's Opera House. He once attended a lecture by Mark Twain. "It was one and a half hours long, but I heard it all and it was mighty good," he noted. When not recording the daily temperature and weather swings in Virginia City, assisting physician, recording the ins and outs of daily life, and tending to his mining interests, Doten enjoyed "drinking cocktails and cruising about town" with his friends, Keyzer and Dan DeQuille, editor of the *Territorial Enterprise*: "Aug. 22, 1866: "This PM, I assisted Dr. Hiller to operate on a leg of John Tookey or Tuohig, which was broken in the Ophir mine some five weeks ago. Dr. [Wakeman] Bryarly has had the case and not doing well was discharged and Dr. Hiller sent for—right leg broken near the ankle–we examined and found leg not set at all–but out of place–we sawed off end of 'tibia,' and picked out lots of small pieces, five or six–Sawed off about an inch–set leg in Iron frame prepared for it, fixed up and left it–took just two hours to do the job–may lose leg yet–very bad job to undertake–All done under chloroform."

Premier Issue, Winter 1989

Vol. XXII, No. 1, Spring 2011

PHYSICIAN AND CONCHOLOGIST

Dr. John Veatch

John Allen Veatch was born on March 5, 1808, the first of eight children in a growing frontier family. In 1822, his mother died, and the family moved to Spencer County, Indiana. At nineteen he was back in Kentucky where he began his medical studies, and it is thought he got his diploma by studying under a practicing doctor.

Unfortunately, we do not have definitive information about his training. Two years later in 1829, his restless nature led him to Louisiana, where he taught school and had two children with his first wife, Charlotte Sheridan (also Edwards).

In 1834, the family moved to Texas where Dr. Veatch acquired land and became involved in politics. He was elected delegate from the Community of Bevil to the Consultation of 1835, which met to consider autonomous rule for Texas a year before the

Texas Declaration of Independence. In the 1840s, Veatch practiced medicine in Town Bluff, Texas. During 1846-47 he served as first lieutenant in the Independent Volunteer Company, and later he served as surgeon in the Texas Mounted Volunteers. After Charlotte's death, Dr. Veatch married Ann Bradley and they had two children. By 1850, he had acquired property and his intellectual interests led him to the study botany and mineralogy. By all accounts Dr. Veatch was a brilliant man. Veatch also once owned what would become some of the most valuable land in Texas at Sour Lake and Spindletop, where oil was discovered.

Still restless for adventure he went to California, and Ann sued for divorce on the basis of abandonment. During his explorations in California, Veatch discovered borax in Lake County. He explored and surveyed Carros Island off Lower California, was curator of conchology at the California Academy of Sciences from 1858 to 1861, and authored several scientific papers.

The Comstock Lode discovery of June 1859 drew Dr. Veatch to the mining district, where he practiced medicine and was involved in geology from 1862 to 1863. He was a resident of Clifton, Lander County in 1863. In 1865 he married his third wife, Samanthe Brisbee, and moved to Oregon. After an unsuccessful attempt to become state geologist of Oregon in 1868 he took a position as professor of chemistry, toxicology, and materia medica at the newly founded Willamette University Medical School. Willamette was Oregon's first medical school, and in 1913 it became the Univ. of Oregon School of Medicine.

Dr. Veatch died of pneumonia in Portland on April 24, 1870. His obituary listed him as an officer of the Ancient United Order of Druids.

EDITORS' NOTE:

Every once in a while, information is brought to our attention about early healthcare in Nevada or in the territory that included the later State of Nevada. Such was the case when Guy Rocha contacted us for information about Dr. John Veatch. He had received an inquiry from Denise Cervantes, Dr. Veatch and Charlotte's (Sheridan) great-great-great-granddaughter. We had information that Veatch was in Nevada in the early 1860s. Denise provided us with a sketch of Dr. Veatch and a biography of him from *The Handbook of Texas Online*.

Vol. XVIII, No. 3, Fall 2007

CHAPTER VIII:
TWENTIETH-CENTURY DOCTORS

In 1901, red cell blood types were discovered, and transfusions would become the wave of the future. Water treated with chlorine to eliminate major bacterial diseases was introduced. Vaccinations against tuberculosis and smallpox eliminated these infections from the 'killer list' of Americans. A most important discovery in 1928 was penicillin, an antibiotic to combat infectious diseases. Its success became prominent during WWII when for the first time doctors treated soldiers successfully for battlefield infections.

By the 1950s, the life expectancy of Americans had increased from less than forty years in 1880 to sixty-five years. In the 1960s. renal dialysis and drugs to treat high blood pressure were introduced, which reduced death from kidney disease, coronary artery disease and cerebral vascular strokes. According to the World Health Organization, numerous discoveries have advanced today's life expectancy of men to over seventy-six years and women to over eighty-one. Prominent advances resulted from early detection and prevention of disease complications and changes in life style, such as reduction in tobacco use. We will not try to enumerate all of the advances, but we assure the reader that we are living in the 'Golden Age of Medicine' as demonstrated by the increase in life expectancy. It is hard to believe that the life expectancy will continue to go up over the next one hundred years at the same rate that it has since 1880. Unfortunately, your authors will not be here to witness the event—if it occurs!

GREAT CARLIN CANYON TRAIN WRECK

Leslie A. Moren MD, Oral History by Owen Bolstad MD

It must have been just after 10:30 pm on the evening of August 12, 1939, because I can remember that the folks were just coming out of the movie theater, when we got the word that there had been a train wreck on the Southern Pacific Railroad, west of Elko. The wreck involved S.P.'s streamliner, *City of San Francisco*, which had roared through Elko westbound only an hour or so earlier.

I had only been in practice in Elko for about a year, having graduated from the University of Minnesota in 1938, so I really hadn't had very much experience in the care of trauma patients. As the youngest man in the group of Hood, Roantree and Secor, I was on weekend call as usual. Dr. Roantree was on vacation that week, so we were already shorthanded.

Dr. A.J. Hood, Tom Hood's father, called me by telephone informing me of the accident, and asked me to assemble whatever emergency supplies and equipment I could gather together and meet him at the railroad station in Carlin (twenty-one miles west of

Elko) where a relief train was being made up, since the site of the wreck could not be reached by road. I really didn't know just what supplies to bring along, but took my stethoscope, a sphygmomanometer, morphine and lots of bandages, together with some bass wood splint material which turned out to be very useful. We all carried flashlights.

In Carlin, I met Dr. Hood and Dr. Fred Poulson, who was another young physician practicing in Elko. Dr. Charles Secor, the senior member of our group, stayed in Elko to care for things there. The relief train, which had been assembled in Carlin, consisted of a number of cabooses, pulled behind the locomotive. It had to proceed westward on the eastbound track, since the westbound tracks had been blocked by the wreckage. The eastbound tracks lay about one fourth of a mile away from the wreck at the nearest point, so we had to walk cross-country in the dark to reach the scene.

The situation at the site of the wreck was horrifying. The derailment had occurred just as the train was crossing a trestle across the Humboldt River. Fourteen of the train's seventeen cars had left the tracks, with Pullman cars strewn everywhere—on their sides, up-ended, across the tracks and in the canyon. The 'dub car' was lying on its side, partially submerged in the river.

The impression that remains etched in my memory now, some fifty years later, is that of the darkness lit only by the feeble light of a few flashlights, and the silence broken only by distant moans and cries for help. I remember a young woman dressed in a pretty blue gown. Both of her legs were gone, and she had long since exsanguinated. Crossing the river, I remember seeing the arm of a porter wearing a white jacket protruding from a window of the 'dub' car. He was trapped beneath the waters of the river and was, of course, dead of drowning.

We did whatever we could at the scene, bandaging wounds, splinting fractures, and administering opiates. With the help of many volunteers from Elko and Carlin, we extricated the injured from the wreckage and carried them to the relief train for transport to the Elko General Hospital and more definitive care. The choice of the caboose cars for the relief train was a poor one, for when we tried to carry the litter onto the cabooses, we found that the safety railings on the ends of the cars made it necessary to negotiate a sharp ninety degree turn into the door at the end of the car.

Twenty-three persons were pronounced dead, and sixty-nine injured passengers were transported to Elko for care. Since the hospital had only had fifty-two beds, and thirty-five beds were already occupied, it was necessary to put many of the injured on spare beds and mattresses in the hallways. A surgeon from San Francisco, Dr. Ward, who was visiting friends in the Elko area, volunteered his help, and the operating room was kept busy for some twenty-four hours. As I recall, we only lost one patient after arriving at the hospital. I think that one was a person with crushing injuries of the chest who could not be stabilized. Not too bad a record for a bunch of county doctors!

The locomotive engineer, who survived the wreck, reported that the train had been travelling at about 70 mph when the accident occurred. He had walked from the scene to get assistance, which accounted for a delay of almost one hour before help was sent. Investigators later determined that a missing tie plate caused the accident, and the Federal Bureau of Investigation stated that it had been an act of sabotage. To this day (2014) no one has been arrested for the crime. Two jackets were found near the scene and were thought to be from the culprits.

Vol. I, No. 3, Fall 1990

FALLON CLINIC
DING, CAFFY, SI, LEN, AND CONNIE

Roderick D. Sage MD

ONE HUNDRED DOCTOR YEARS

The nicknames Ding, Caffy, Si, Len, and Connie rekindle fond memories of the much-loved quintet of physicians who served the Nevada area surrounding Fallon for upwards of one hundred doctor years. Dr. Alphonse J. Dingacci was universally known as 'Ding' to his many patients and friends. Dr. Darius Caffaratti logically went by 'Caffy.' Dr. Verlyn Elliott was known as 'Si,' a moniker he acquired in childhood. Dr. Leonard Miller was simply 'Len.' These medical practitioners were the sum and substance of the Fallon Clinic from 1949 to the early 1990s. Dr. Dingacci, and his friend and colleague, Dr. Leonard Miller, had worked together in Hawthorne, Nevada, before coming to Fallon where, in due time, they collaborated on organizing and building the Fallon Clinic, which opened its doors in January 1949. They left their offices on Auction Road near the old hospital to move into the 4,000 square foot, up-to-date structure at the corner of Taylor Street and Williams Avenue.

DR. DARIUS CAFFARATTI

Caffy's life began in Italy in 1916, but at the age of two he came to San Jose, California with his family.

After prep school at Bellarmire Academy, he attended Santa Clara, where he became Ding's roommate and lifelong friend. Caffy graduated from St. Louis University Medical School in 1941, his academic career having been capped by selection for membership in Phi Beta Kappa at Santa Clara and Alpha Omega Alpha at St. Louis University. These are well-respected undergraduate and medical scholastic honor societies.

Caffy, whose lifelong hearing impairment excluded him from the service, started his career as director of a tuberculosis hospital in Oroville, California. He followed this with two years of work as a resident physician and clinician at the Butte County Hospital in Oroville. Then in 1946 he launched his own family practice in that northern California community where he served for eighteen years.

Caffy left Oroville in 1962 for a year of European travel with his family. He used this opportunity to obtain more medical training in Vienna and London. Returning to the United States in 1963, Dr. Caffaratti contacted his old friend, Ding, and promptly became an associate in the Fallon Clinic.

Darius Caffaratti was dark complexioned, compact, and loquacious. His many opinions about life in general, and especially medicine, were expressed with his quite distinctively rasp-like voice. In the 1960 presidential election, while still in Oroville, Caffy managed the regional campaign for Jack Kennedy, but in due time abandoned the Democratic Party to become a staunch Republican. He was an avowed enemy of socialized medicine, worked to legalize prostitution in Churchill County and served as the Churchill County Public Health Officer.

Caffy was an inveterate collector of old cars, cameras, swords, and firearms. He had his own photographic dark room in addition to a wood working shop. He excelled artistically in both endeavors. After 18 years with the Fallon Clinic, Caffy died quite suddenly in September 1981 leaving wife Rose, daughter Barbara, now an internist in Portland, Oregon, and son John, a cardiologist in Ohio.

DR. ALPHONSE J. DINGACCI

Ding was born in 1915 in San Mateo, California. After high school there he graduated from Santa Clara University in 1937 and Creighton University School of Medicine in Omaha in 1941.

Ding was an avid duck hunter and knew the Greenhead Club intimately. He was also an accomplished musician with special abilities on the accordion, clarinet, and organ. Though his wife, Pat, was an excellent horsewoman, Ding shunned this sport, but was regularly the attending physician at the area rodeos. Ding was a small and wiry man, possessed of a mischievous twinkle in his eye and an enviable sense of humor.

Both Caffaratti and Dingacci returned to Santa Clara County Hospital for their internships. Ding continued for two more years of surgical training after which he served as an army surgeon in Europe until discharged in 1946.

DR. VERLYN (SI) ELLIOTT

Si Elliott was born in 1924 and grew up in eastern South Dakota. He served in World War II as a navy radioman, then, returned for premed at Yankton College. He completed the two-year medical curriculum at the University of South Dakota, then, obtained his MD degree from Colorado University in Denver in 1952. Si interned at the Public Health Service Hospital in San Francisco, then went on to the Walker River Indian Service Hospital in Schurz, Nevada, for three years, followed by a stint of general practice and employment with Kennecott Corporation in Ely. In 1958, he joined Ding at the Fallon Clinic.

In contrast to his clinic partners, Si Elliott was somewhat angular of build, quiet, and taciturn by nature. A caring and attentive physician, he became active in medical politics, eventually serving as president of the nsma in 1970-71. He followed this with a term on the Medical Board of Examiners. Si and his wife Joan raised four children in Fallon, the oldest of whom served in the navy as a MD. His hobbies included training horses at their ranch on the outskirts of Fallon. He enjoyed duck and deer hunting, but especially each autumn, he savored a trek to his native South Dakota for pheasant shooting. He was also the team physician for many of the Fallon high school sports activities.

In 1976, Si moved from Fallon to a new practice in Reno. The following year he suffered a severely disabling stroke, which forced him to retire from medicine completely. He died in 1990 at sixty-six.

Dr. Leonard Miller

The fourth member of this group, Dr. Leonard Miller, had practiced with Dr. Dingacci for two years in the late 1940s, and helped to establish the Fallon Clinic. He stayed until 1953 at which time he entered a three-year psychiatry residency program, variously in Mexico, Hawaii, and New York City.

Dr. Miller, a native of Kansas, was born in 1912, acquired the necessary schooling there, and then, was awarded an MD degree from Kansas University in 1938. He interned in Detroit, did general practice in Dodge City, Kansas, and then, worked for the Civilian Conservation Corp. in California before becoming a navy doctor. He ultimately was the medical officer for mine sweepers in the Pacific theater.

Len practiced psychiatry in San Francisco for eighteen years where he did research on substance abuse problems at the University of California and California Medical Facility in Vacaville. For two years in the 1960s Len Miller demonstrated his free and independent spirit by living in (or out of) a van on the side of Mt. Tamalpais in Marin County, sleeping under the stars, then going about his necktie and white coat doctor role during the day.

In 1975, Dr. Miller pulled up stakes again, heading 300 miles east, to God's Country–Fallon, Nevada–where he rejoined the Fallon Clinic, which he had left twenty-two years earlier.

Len was a man of medium size, sturdily built, and with a sartorial elegance akin to that of Buffalo Bill Cody.

Between them the four doctors treated well over one hundred patients daily in the clinic. They made hospital rounds once or twice a day and many house calls. Their scheduling allowed one doctor to be off for periods of five days, while night calls were rotated amongst the others. This amounted to a workweek of 60 to 90 hours per physician. They needed those five free days just to recover.

Dr. Conrad Frydenlund

After serving as a bombardier in World War II, flying fifty-two missions, and being a prisoner of war for nine months, Dr. Conrad Frydenlund finished medical school at the University of Minnesota in 1951, followed by a year of internship at San Bernardino County Hospital. After briefly practicing in Minnesota, he returned west to Reno, being employed for three months as a clinic doctor for Washoe Hospital. At this juncture he learned that Dr. Dingacci needed an associate to replace the departed Dr. Len Miller.

Connie's proposed short locum tenens stretched into an eight-year stint with the Fallon Clinic. On his second day in Fallon he was called to attend an elderly sick woman in Hazen, fifteen miles to the west. He found, to his consternation, a badly bloated and decomposed corpse of an old woman lying in a shack, half buried in filthy blankets. Soon after that he delivered six babies in one day, and made the first of several house calls to Austin, one hundred miles east. That's jumping in with both feet.

Dr. Frydenlund left Fallon in 1961 to pursue a radiology residency in Santa Monica and practiced in that city. He retired to Saline, Michigan, at seventy-eight.

Dr. Gary Ridenour

Dr. Gary Ridenour joined the Fallon Clinic in 1984. The most recent member of the Fallon Clinic doctors, he grew up in Cleveland, matriculated at Hiram College in Ohio, and then earned his MD degree at the University of Guadalajara in Mexico in 1978. He followed this with an intern year at St. Louis University and came to Fallon in 1980. He practiced solo for a year, and then joined the clinic. He submits a telling record of his experience with Dr. Dingacci and a fascinating commentary on his maturing as a young doctor.

Dr. Ridenour relates:

"On my first day with Dr. Dingacci he showed me my office. I sat down in the swivel chair at the desk. As I rocked back, I immediately flipped over."

Ding chuckled and said:

"Watch that chair, Gary. Dr. Caffaratti once got a subdural from it."

"The next day it was fixed. When I first came to Fallon, I was a hot doctor from the East, and Ding took me into his practice. I thought I was doing a good job, but Ding had a very dedicated following. I then began to appreciate that Ding sat down and simply visited with his patients, obtaining more information about their ailments than I ever did.

Ding:

"If you really listen to the patient, they will tell you what is wrong with them. Never be arrogant and never get mad. They are paying for a service and expect a little more than you popping into a room, then popping out. If you want to get rich, go into business. If you want to be happy, do what I do."

Dr. Ridenour:

"I chose happy, I hadn't worn cowboy boots for years, when I noticed Ding's alligator boots and told him I liked them."

Ding noted:

"They are comfortable easy to get on in the middle of the night, and you don't have to wear socks."

Dr. Ridenour:

"I have worn boots since then, but usually with socks. When I first went to the store with Ding, everyone said Hello. I frowned and said, "I don't have to be their friend, just their doctor."

Ding frowned back and observed: "In a small town, you are a big part of it and not invisible. Get used to it. It's fun."

Dr. Ridenour: "I once complained to Ding that some of his elderly patients were 'crocks' with not much wrong with them."

Ding smiled: "They are all alone and scared of dying. They look forward to coming to us. It's our job to help them."

Dr. Ridenour: "I was once surprised when Ding, with a sly grin, greeted an elderly woman with, "Well you old bat, what's wrong this time?" The old lady smiled and began her story."

Ding explained: "Making fun of getting old was good therapy, Getting old is something we all have in common, and we should not let it get us down."

Dr. Ridenour concludes: "Of all the doctors I have known and learned from, Ding was head and shoulders above the rest. When he didn't know something, he asked other doctors. He earned a spot in my heart as a kind, gentle, and caring man. Give 'em Hell in Heaven, Ding!"

THANK YOU, DOCTORS

In 1987, Dr. Dingacci retired from his medical practice. At the same time he was named Emeritus Clinical Professor of the University of Nevada School of Medicine. Pat and Ding found a winter haven in Arizona where they basked in the warm winter sunshine, while learning the intricacies of the game of golf. Summers were spent amongst their many friends back in Fallon.

Ding's later retirement years were tragically disrupted by a severe neurologic injury he suffered in a fall from a pickup truck while helping to prepare a barbecue supper. Though confined to a wheelchair, his spirits remained indomitable until the end of his life at eighty-eight in 2004.

Dr. Miller maintained a part-time practice until the early 1990s, eventually succumbing in 1995 at the age of eighty-two.

Vol. XV, No. 3, Winter 2004

EDITORS' NOTE:

Doctors Kurt Carlson and Tim Hockenberry were valued colleagues, but not members of the Fallon Clinic. Bunny Corkill of the Churchill County Museum and Archives and Willi Whomes, former chief nurse of the Churchill Public Hospital added information on the clinic. Dr. Jack Flanary of Reno was stationed at Fallon Air Station where he knew Dr. Frydenlund in the 1950s and brought him to our attention.

WOMEN'S RIGHTS ADVOCATE
Dr. Eliza Cook

Dr. Eliza Cook was a pillar of strength in her community and a respected member of the medical profession. Her life represents a transition between the 19th and 20th-century practice of medicine in Nevada. Her story begins in 19th-century England, where her parents initially lived. They later converted to the Mormon faith and moved to Utah. Eliza was born in Salt Lake City on February 5, 1856, but the family moved several times before finally settling in the Carson Valley in 1870.

The first two decades of her life were spent helping her family make ends meet. She and her sister worked for neighboring families, helping with household chores. There was no school in her Carson Valley community, so she borrowed books from neighbors and was self-taught. At the age of twenty-three, Eliza nursed Dr. H.W. Smith's wife, who had post-partum complications. This two-year endeavor gave her time to read medical books in Dr. Smith's library, and he encouraged her to study medicine. Eliza spent six months apprenticing under Dr. Smith before she pursued her medical education in San Francisco at Cooper Medical College. Eliza graduated in 1884 with four other women in a class of sixteen. (The first woman to graduate from an American medical school was Elizabeth Blackwell, who graduated from Geneva Medical College in New York in 1848.) Dr. Cook settled in Markleeville for a short time before attending Women's Medical College of Philadelphia and the Medical College of New York.

In 1891, she returned to Nevada and practiced in Reno for a few months, but the appeal of the Carson Valley was too great. She built a home in Mottsville and spent the rest of her career there. Dr. Cook never married and was a lifelong active supporter of women's rights and the Women's Christian Temperance Union. She was a leader in the organization and served as president for five years. Dr. Cook practiced medicine until she retired at the age of sixty-five. In recognition of her contributions to medicine, the waiting room in the first Carson-Tahoe Hospital was named the Eliza Cook Room.

She died at the age of 91 in her home. Although Dr. Cook was inaccurate when she said, "As far as I know I was the first woman to practice in Nevada," she had another distinction. Guy Rocha stated, "Dr. Eliza Cook did what female doctors before her did not do. She lived and died in Nevada."

Vol. III, No. 1, Summer 1992

NEVADA'S DOCTOR FOR THE AGES
DR. MARY FULSTONE

Anton P. Sohn MD

Dr. Mary Fulstone graduated from an allopathic medical school, the University of California in San Francisco. The year 1920 was in the interval between wwi and ii. Unfortunately, women were still felt by many to be unable to carry out the physical demands required of a physician and surgeon. Mary Hill did not accept this verdict and became a doctor.

Her life began in 1892 in Eureka, Nevada, and in 1896 she moved to Carson City with her family. At Carson High School, she excelled in academics and athletics and was interested in outdoor activities, but after graduation in 1911, she pursued her ambition to become a physician. She attended the University of California in Berkeley and graduated from its medical school in San Francisco in 1917. After two years of postgraduate training at Children's Hospital and the San Francisco County Hospital, she married Fred Fulstone and returned to Nevada to practice in Smith Valley.

Dr. Mary's practice in Smith Valley spanned sixty-five years and her leadership in the community and state is legendary. She was a leader who got things done, and she led the Lyon County Hospital into the modern era by obtaining Hill-Burton government funds to modernize and enlarge the hospital. By her personality and influence, she was able to persuade leading doctors in Reno to be on the hospital staff and provide consultation services.

She raised a family of five children. Dr. Mary found time to devote her considerable talents in service to the community. In 1916, she was named 'Nevada Mother of the Year,' in 1963, nsma named her 'The Physician of the Year,' and in 1964 the Univ. of Nev. honored her as 'The Distinguished Citizen of the Year.' She served on the State Board of Education and Smith Valley Board of Education.

The 1940s saw changes in women's place in society. WWII thrust them into the workplace, and they demonstrated that they had the physical attributes and endurance to work alongside men in industrial and medical professions. Nevertheless, little changed for women's rights until the 1960s and '70s when equal rights for race became headlines in the nation. The assassination of Dr. Martin Luther King pierced the heart of America, and things began to change. The Vietnam War protest was the spark that lit the fire signifying that Americans wanted a change in government policy. Later, the U.S. Government passed Title IX in 1979, which changed the nation's athletic scene by forcing equal funding for women in sports.

At the same time a quiet revolution was taking place in medicine as medical schools were admitting more women. Furthermore, dramatic advances were occurring in electronic technology and treatment of disease. Thus, medicine was launched into the modern era and women became a large part of it.

XVI, No. 2, Summer 2005

ADVENTURES OF A COUNTRY DOCTOR

Oral History by Mary Ellen Glass

I was married my last year when I was (in medical school) in San Francisco, and then I came up here and moved to this house and have been here ever since, fifty-three years. When I came up here it was kind of nice because they'd never had a doctor here before. So there was no discrimination between a woman and a man doctor. They were so—I think they were so happy to have a doctor right in the community; they'd had to send to Yerington for their doctors before. And to know that was a horse and buggy drive up here, which was kind of long, arid they had all gone through that influenza epidemic without having a doctor here. I think they were very happy, because there were a good many deaths and very serious illnesses, and they were happy to have one. But of course, there were probably some who think, "Oh, a woman doctor, how terrible!"

But I always said the Indian people were my saviors. They took to me right away; that is, they were going to try me out right away. So many of them worked on our ranch right here. In those days, before they had the new machinery, you know, you'd have twenty men working, where maybe now there'd be five. And they all came and got little things— cuts and bruises and sickness, so they took to me right away and I always said, "Well, I think they were good advertisers." (Laughing) And I have been very friendly with the Indians, with the Indian population here throughout the years.

Have (had) lots of funny experiences. I was even asked to consult with an Indian medicine man at one time, which was quite an idea. I went up here to the camp and walked in and the room was all decorated, you know, in different things, like little feathers and a little bow and arrow and things like that all around. The patient had a little band on her head and a feather or two up. And we had a consultation, the Indian medicine man and I did. He said, "Well, I thought might be well to consult with you because I could help you a little bit by telling you what the Indians took as laxatives and things like that, you know."

And I said, "Oh, I think you could, you'll be a great help." We had quite a little conversation. Come to find out, he was an Indian man that had worked on this very ranch and just lately had gone into being an Indian medicine man.

In the beginning I used to go to Bridgeport, Coleville, Sweetwater, and all around. In fact, I had a contract for a while with the government in taking care of those patients.

But one little story—I went up to Sweetwater one night to deliver a baby. They said this woman was having a great deal of trouble having her baby. Indians usually didn't have a doctor when they had their children; they seemed to get along all right. But this baby was a cross presentation and an arm had come down in the deliverance area. The other Indian woman had been pulling on the arm, you know, thinking if they pulled hard enough they'd get the baby out, not realizing that they couldn't do it. So finally they sent for me. The baby was dead, of course, but I went up. It was—we'd been away 'someplace and had just come back; it was quite late in the night Fred drove me up, and here she was in a little tent, you know, right on their little beds (which) were always on the floor. So we had to get one of the neighbors up and get a kitchen table and get her up on that. So I had one Indian woman giving a few drops of ether to kind of ease off the pain, two other Indian women kind of assisting me. The two Indian women kept saying, "Now Mary, you wouldn't leave us would you? You're going to stay here aren't you?"

And I said, "No, I wouldn't leave." The sweat was rolling down; I was working hard. The other Indian woman kept saying, "Do you think you can make it; do you think you're going to get the baby; do you think you can make it?" So finally, anyway, after quite a long siege, I got the baby delivered and the woman back in her bed and comfortable. I was just terrified that surely she'd have an infection, you know, up there with nothing very sterile. But she got better. Finally, about 2 months later, we were having dinner out here and there was a rap on the door of my office and the housekeeper went. She opened the door and there was a big, tall Indian there and she says, "Oh, you want to see Dr. Mary."

He says, "No, I want to see Fred." And so Fred went to the door and the Indian man said, "Oh, hello, Fred," and Fred said, "Hello." He says, "Oh, Fred, your wife came up and took care of my wife and now she's all better and I've come down to pay you. Now what do you charge?" (*Laughing*)

EDITORS' NOTE:

Reference: Oral history conducted for the UN Library by Mary Ellen Glass, between July 5, 1973 and Feb. 7, 1974. The title is "Recollections of a Country Doctor in Smith, Nev."

Vol. I, No. 4, Winter 1990-91

RESEARCHER AND EPIDEMIOLOGIST
Dr. Sandra Daugherty

Sandra Keller was born June 27, 1934, in Kansas City, Missouri. Sandra began her career at the University of Kansas where she earned an undergraduate degree in Music and Literature in 1956 and her MD in 1960. She was one of four women (3.8 percent) in a class of one hundred and five. Sandra also sang in the University of Kansas Chorale as a freshman medical student, the only medical student who had ever done so. During her second year of medical school, her talent earned her an audition with the Metropolitan Opera.

She earned a PhD in public health at the University of Oklahoma and took a residency in public health and preventive medicine. Her academic career took her from Oklahoma to Michigan State where she was the first woman in the country to be the principal investigator of a National Institutes of Health (NIH) clinical trial. She worked from 1971 to 1976 on the Hypertension Detection and Follow-up Program, a national study that led to the awareness that physicians need to treat high blood pressure more actively. Her successful work on blood pressure earned her and her colleagues a prestigious Special Public Health Award from the Lasker Foundation in 1980.

During her career, Dr. Daugherty was the recipient of more than $20 million in peer-reviewed funding from the nih. In 1995, she was responsible for securing the largest grant ever awarded to the UN System—$8.5 million for the Women's Health Initiative. She investigated the effects of various treatments on the reduction of death among patients with high blood pressure and other forms of heart disease. In addition, she studied mercury levels in Dayton, Nevada, and its effects on residents' health. She conducted an epidemiological study of chronic fatigue syndrome at Lake Tahoe, concluding that it is, in fact, a disease, and not a psychological malady as many physicians thought.

Dr. Daugherty spent many years working with the National Heart, Lung and Blood Institute and the American Heart Association on review committees, study sections, and conference planning committees. She was one of the first women to assume a leadership role with the American Heart Association, where she served on the Executive Committee and as chair of the Council on Epidemiology. Dr. Daugherty was on the University of Nevada School of Medicine faculty for nineteen years and was the first woman to earn the rank of professor. She died May 31, 2000.

Vol. XI, No. 4, Winter 2000-01

WOMEN DOCTORS
IN TWENTIETH-CENTURY NEVADA

Anton P. Sohn MD

The aamcs' statistics show that women comprised 5.7 percent of medical school graduates in 1959; the percentages slightly increased to 8.4 in 1969; and jumped up to 32.1 percent in 1979 and 34.5 percent in 1989. In 2005 equality was achieved.

GRADUATES OF NEVADA'S MEDICAL SCHOOL

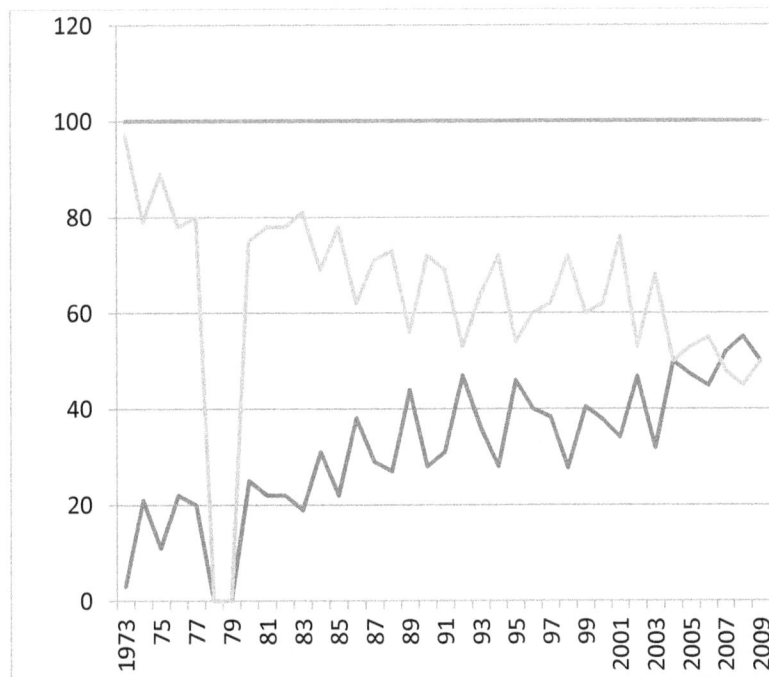

The upper curve is the percent of male graduates.
The lower curve is the percent of female graduates.
Between 1978 and 1980 the School went to a four-year program.

CALL IN INDIAN COUNTRY
DR. JAMES W. GEROW

Lynn Gerow, Sr. MD

One morning, my father (Dr. James Wiggins Gerow, was awakened by a persistently ringing telephone. On the other end was the Indian agent from Nixon. Nevada, saying that one of the Winnemucca squaws was about to have a baby—could he come immediately. How my father had any responsibility for treating Indians. I do not know. However, it seems that went with the position of Washoe County Physician. All the Indians in the county thought of him as chief medicine man and every Indian in the area knew him on a first name basis. That name was "Doc." There were many good friends in the area's Indian nation.

Dad quietly awakened me and asked if I would like to help him deliver an Indian baby. I sprang out of bed as eager as if it was the first day of fishing season. While I dressed and had a hurried breakfast, Dad was in the garage 'steaming up' his Stanley Steamer for the trip.

The Steamer was a long black seven passenger open riding car that moved along with ease at any speed. It emitted only a hissing noise along with a small amount of white steam through its exhaust. On cold days the steam was much more evident, and the car would sometimes appear to be a white cloud as it silently moved through traffic. One of the notable things about the car was that it fit my father's sense of humor. The car developed a charge of static electricity when it was being steamed up to a head of pressure sufficient to move the large pistons. If a person was in the car, he would not notice the electricity generated but, if one was standing on the ground and touched the car or put his foot on the running board, he would get a charge of static electricity that would make all the hairs on his head standup.

Many times I was in the car while the boiler was being steamed and someone would pass by making smart remarks about the steam buggy. My father would call out, "Hey. George, come here a minute." When the wisecracker came over he would put his foot on the running board to hear what Dad had to tell him all his hair would stand on end. A shocked expression would appear which was always followed by ugly blasphemy and a loud chuckle by my father. Soon everyone in town knew it was dangerous to touch "Old Stanley" at such a time.

After an hour and a half drive, we arrived at Nixon. The Indian agent directed us to an 8' x 12' white army tent. On entering we found a young squaw lying on a deer hide obviously in labor. Her "*Aye, Yi, Yis*" were heard throughout the camp with each labor pain. Surrounding her were four older squaws administering to her needs with cool sips of water, fanning with a chafing fan, giving words of encouragement and going, "*Aye, Yi. Yis*" with her every contraction.

My father cleared the tent of all but one squaw and me. Following an examination to determine the stage of labor, she was given 'Twilight Sleep' and prepared for delivery. During the next forty minutes and many subdued, "*Aye, Yi, Yis.*" Dad remarked, "Do you smell something burning?" He directed me out of the tent to investigate. About fifty yards away the ground was mounded up along a thirty-foot long trench and smoke was coming up through the soil. It smelled something like burning hair and fat.

Several bucks were in attendance, but they were unable to tell me what was going on. Back to the maternity ward I went. Giving Dad a report, he retorted, "Burning garbage, I guess." At that moment the baby's head came into view and a yelling baby girl was brought into the world to a happy mother. Following delivery of the after-birth, the squaws were summoned into the tent to attend the needs of mother and child, which they did with much chatter and deliberation.

After leaving the tent, we were met by a group of happy men who told us they had been preparing a feast to celebrate the occasion. Directing us to the smoldering pit, we saw the men unearthing dozens of smoking, steaming *Puldoos*. *Puldoos* are mud hens. These particular birds had not been dressed. The feathers remained on the skin, the entrails were in the body cavities, and the heads and webbed feet were still present. The master of ceremonies insisted we remain for dinner to celebrate the arrival of the new princess. My father tactfully declined, stating that there was another woman in labor in Reno who needed his attention. They accepted this explanation. The old Stanley was steamed up to half a head and we made a hasty getaway down the country road.

About two weeks later, a committee of Indians brought my father a gift of appreciation. There were seven arrows, the shafts made of tagemite (a reed which grows wild along the Truckee River), colorful goose feather flyers, and beautiful obsidian points. Appreciation was gratefully shown, and the committee returned to Nixon.

These arrows were later given to Dorothy Smith, wife of Harold Smith, Sr., who displayed them in Harold's Club for a number of years. Mrs. Smith has since returned them to me and they remain as one of my most cherished possessions, recalling one of my most pleasant and exciting memories.

EDITORS' NOTE:

- This story about his father, Dr. James Wiggins Gerow, was related by the late Dr. Lynn Gerow, Sr. in his autobiography, *First Opinion,* an unpublished manuscript given to us by his son, Dr. Lynn Gerow, Jr. The manuscript contains many other fascinating stories about life and the practice of medicine in the early years. Some of these may appear in later issues of *GWT.*

- James Gerow was born in California in 1879 and received his MD from California Medical College in San Francisco in 1902. He was licensed in Sparks, Nevada, in 1905 and died in Reno April 9, 1951. His son, Lynn, Sr., was a family practitioner, and grandson, Lynn Jr., a psychiatrist, practiced in Reno.

Vol. II, No. 2, Summer 1991

ADVENTURE IN THE HIGH SIERRA
DR. LAURENCE NELSON

Oral History by Owen Bolstad MD

During the winter of 1951-52 a fierce storm hit the Sierra Nevada It snowed heavily for almost a month. Winds of over 100 mph were recorded at Donner Summit and the temperature was near zero. Drifting snow had completely blocked U.S. Highway #40. The little town of Truckee, California, had been snowbound for some time.

On Sunday morning January 13, 1952, the westbound streamliner *City of San Francisco,* an extra fare luxury train carrying 226 passengers plus its crew, became stalled by an avalanche west of Donner Summit. Many of the passengers aboard the train were delegates to the National Republican Convention, which was to be held in San Francisco the following week. Rescue units with rotary snow plows were dispatched. Rotary plows sent to rescue the train were stalled or broken down. Passengers aboard the snowbound streamliner passed the first night in relative comfort with heat provided by the diesel engines and with plenty of food on board the dining car. There was no panic, and most regarded the adventure as a lark, confident that they would soon be rescued.

On Monday afternoon Dr. Laurence D. Nelson, was asked if he would try to reach the scene to assist those aboard, and Nelson readily agreed to try. After a brief prayer Nelson donned his winter clothing, grabbed his medical bag and set out.

An ambitious twenty-nine-year-old, healthy and confident, he felt up to the challenge. He went into Truckee and contacted Lloyd VanSykle, a well-known dogsled racer. VanSykle agreed to help him, and soon they boarded a locomotive and steamed up the grade to Norden. They unloaded the rig in the Norden tunnel, and assembled the team and sled. With Dr. Nelson snugly tucked into the vehicle they started out. Moments after they emerged from the tunnel into the fury of the blizzard, the lead dog completely disappeared into the deep powdery snow. Soon the entire team was floundering about in the powder, and it became apparent that proceeding by dog sled was impossible.

Dr. Nelson then set out alone by snowshoe, passing Soda Springs to reach Donner Summit Lodge. With snow so deep that the entrance to the lodge was blocked, he entered the lodge on the third-floor level, and stopped there to rest and have a bite to eat. Reevaluating his situation over a cup of coffee, he decided to snowshoe down U.S. Highway #40. By then, dusk had fallen. Huge drifts surrounded the road, and overhanging cornices of snow threatened to avalanche at any time. Along the highway there were tall stands of Ponderosa pine that protected the road from winds. Larry relates that, at times, the moonlight would break through the clouds revealing a scene of incredible beauty around him. He describes an awesome silence, broken only by the rustle of wind in the tops of the tall pines.

Trudging on through the night he became increasingly fatigued, and at one point, fell face forward in the powdery snow. With his snowshoes buoying up his feet, and unable to gain any purchase with his hands, he floundered about for some time. He said that he lay there in the snow, warm and comfortable. Realizing how easy it would be to lie there and die peacefully, he renewed his efforts, and finally was able to stand upright and continue the journey.

Continuing throughout the night he arrived at Nyack Lodge at daybreak. Entering the lodge, he had breakfast and slept for several hours. When he awakened, he found that Mr. Jay Gold, a supervisor for Pacific Gas and Electric, was at the lodge. Best of all he had a Sno-Cat that was capable of negotiating the deep snow.

Gold had been working without rest for thirty-six hours ferrying supplies and personnel to and from the site of the stranded train. He agreed to take Dr. Nelson to the scene, and, as they approached the train, Nelson saw an indescribable scene. Huge drifts surrounded the cars and large icicles hung from the corners of the cars. About thirty-five section hands from nearby Crystal Lake were valiantly trying to keep the ventilators beneath the cars clear of snow, and maintain a footpath beside the cars.

Entering the train he met the train master, who briefed him on conditions. Making rounds in the train, he found no serious illnesses. Later, he was approached by one of the Mexican section hands. The man's 1-year-old child was desperately ill at his home in Crystal Lake and needed attention. Although by that time he was completely exhausted, Nelson agreed to see the child. Again he set out on foot for Crystal Lake, some two or three miles distant. He found the child had severe tonsillitis and administered medication. Then he asked for a pillow and a blanket, lay down on the floor and slept for almost eight hours. Returning to the train. \

Dr. Nelson found that the situation there was rapidly becoming tenser. The only food remaining on the train was beans, which were being served at every meal, much to the 'distress' of all on board. The sanitary facilities had been overwhelmed, and conditions were bad in spite of a bucket brigade organized by the train master. The prolonged internment was getting on the nerves of everyone. They began to show increasing symptoms of stress. Nelson, together with the conductor and train master, began to plan for the evacuation of the passengers.

The train was stalled not far from a place where the railroad bridged Highway #101, about five miles from Nyack Lodge. Skies were clear, and winds were calm, so they began detraining the passengers. Group by group they hiked down the path that had been kept open by the section hands, and were driven to Nyack Lodge by five automobiles owned by lodge employees.

There they were fed and cared for until a relief train from San Francisco arrived to transport them to their destination.

Jay Gold, who did such heroic work with the Sno-Cat, was stricken by a massive coronary occlusion brought on by sheer exhaustion. He died on the way to Colfax. Another fatality was recorded when the engineer of one of the rotary snowplow was buried by an overturned engine. The Republicans reached San Francisco in time to attend the convention, and nominate Dwight D. Eisenhower for the presidency of the United States. That November he was elected as our thirty-fourth president.

Vol. II, No. 3, Fall 1991

EDITORS NOTE:

Laurence D. Nelson graduated from Loma Linda som and practiced in Truckee before serving in the U.S. Navy from 1952 to 1954 during the Korean War. After his tour of duty, he returned to Truckee to practice before doing surgical training in San Francisco. Dr. Nelson moved to Sparks, Nevada, in 1968. He served as the Sparks Police Surgeon and died in 1992.

DETAR MEDICAL LEGACY
Doctors Jake, Tom, Jo, Mike, and Ed

Robert M. Daugherty MD

(Father) John 'Jake' DeTar, 86 (Died Nov. 20, 2011)

I knew Urologist John 'Jake' DeTar from afar during my twenty years as dean. For several years, he would write me a very respectful letter strongly suggesting that as dean of the medical school I should not be on the board of Planned Parenthood because he believed they were performing abortions. As I learned over the years, Jake had a fervent belief against abortions. The more I learned about his activities and beliefs, I realized that he and I did not agree; however, I certainly admired and respected his passion for his beliefs. Despite his passion, appreciated the respectful way he disagreed.

I also knew that two of his children were graduated physicians, Jo (1987) and Michael (1989), who attended the University of Nevada School of Medicine during my tenure as dean. I did not know that two additional children, Edward (msu, 1998) and Tom (usc, 1986), also became physicians. Twelve siblings and four physicians! To have a third of one's children become physicians led me to seek out these four siblings and ask what influence their father had on their choices. Below are their responses.

(Son) Tom, Otolaryngologist, Coeur d'Alene

Although I am number eight of twelve, I was the first of the kids to pursue medicine. Both my father and physician grandfather inspired me, but I also have an uncle and cousins who are physicians.

My father kept an extra phone in our house linked to his office, so patients were surprised to hear his voice when they called his office in the evening or weekends. His personal attention to his patients served as a wonderful example to me, as I now call my patients at home after their operations.

I attended unr with a major in premed studies and a minor in German. Dad encouraged me to keep my education as broad as possible, as professional school tends to narrow a mind's perspective. I thank him to this day for such wonderful advice. Reading Virgil, Goethe, and the classics was possible then, but it would be difficult now.

I have always felt it was a privilege to take care of patients, enjoying the challenge of diagnosis, and improving my surgical skills. Perhaps, my enthusiasm for medicine is why my son, Will, is a junior at unr and planning to apply for medical school this coming year, 2013. I have never regretted my decision, and remain indebted to my father and grandfather for showing me the way.

(Daughter) Josephine, Anesthesiologist, Elmira

I went to college, intending on teaching physical education as a career. Of course, along the way, I changed my mind and decided to put my love of physical education and sciences together to become a doctor.

Would I do it again? Most definitely! I have always felt that I had been given a great privilege to be accepted into the medical profession and to receive the mantle of a physician. There have been several times when I know that my involvement in a patient's care has made the difference between living and dying. And I say that those few instances are why I travelled the road I did—just to be there, at that time—and made a difference.

I am also blessed to be able to say I still love my work. I'm not just 'working for the weekend.' So I thank my following mentors, over the years, for making it possible for me to do what I do:

- My father for teaching me how to ski, sail, ride bicycles, for his foresight in our home—no TV—just books from ceiling to floor in every room where a wall was available; for English grammar lessons at the dinner table; for taking us to Mass every Sunday; teaching us about ethics and logic; and handily having a lot of interesting literature lying about the house.
- My teachers: Mr. Riordan, at Bishop Manogue High School; my first grade teacher, Sister Maryanna, sixth grade teacher, Sister Boniface; my chemistry teacher at unr, Mr. Chuck Rose; and Mr. Loper in the physical education department. I also must add Dr. Sohn to my list because he let me come to the coroner's office to watch autopsies, which helped me get into medical school.
- So that's where my path came from and where it led.

(SON) MICHAEL, PATHOLOGIST, COEUR D'ALENE

Our family has a number of physicians, including my father and his father before him, and they certainly played a large role in my decision to pursue medicine.

I recall as a boy attending a ranch style picnic with my father at the home of a long time country doctor, Dr. Mary Fulstone, in Yerington, where I met Dr. Salvadorini, a Reno doctor.

When I later asked my father what kind of doctor he was, he told me he was a pathologist. I didn't know what a pathologist was and queried about that as well. My father responded by describing a pathologist as a, "Doctor's doctor who has to know everything." That seemed like a pretty daunting area of medicine to me, and I didn't really think about pathology again until my second year of medical school, when I studied under Doctors Sohn, Ritzlin, and Malin at UNRSOM .

I have encountered many in medicine who have lost the joy of 'Practicing the Art.' The administrative burden is huge, and the 'compliance' requirements have made the practice of medicine unwieldy and hazardous. Despite these challenges, I consider my choice of specialty to have been a wise and personally rewarding one. When people ask me if I would go through medical school, "If I had to do it all over again," I tell them, "Yes, it was a challenge, but when young, fearless, and foolish, and when 'securing the

prize' seems attainable, the sacrifices are well worth the effort, and I would do it again."
(SON) EDWARD, SURGEON, COEUR D'ALENE

I am the youngest of the twelve John DeTar children and have always felt that my family was very unique and wonderful. I have been blessed to have such a one-of-a-kind father and have so many great older siblings. In fact, I think the uniqueness of my family is perhaps why I am a doctor today.

As a child I always felt drawn to medicine and from my earliest days I recall wanting to be a doctor. I admired what my grandfather, father, and older siblings, and I felt it was the noblest of professions.

I applied to medical school and was granted two interviews. I did well on one and totally bombed the other. Someone from admissions called me a week later and told me that they would like to grant me a third interview since my first 2 were so polarizing. My third interview started off benign, then the interviewer asked me about my family. This led to a one+ hour talk about my family. In the end, she found me, by virtue of my unique family, to be a good candidate and I was accepted.

To this day, I am convinced I was accepted to medical school partially because of my achievements, but mostly because of my unique large family with my one-of-a-kind dad.

I now practice general surgery and vascular surgery with 5 partners. I thoroughly enjoy my practice and cannot imagine doing anything else. I am in my ninth year since finishing residency and feel today as I did at age 13, that medicine is a noble profession, every day is fascinating, and there is nothing I would rather be doing.

EDITORS' NOTE:

Dr. Jake DeTar very much influenced four of his twelve children to enter the profession of Medicine, not only as a caring father, but he was in many ways their physician role model. A true family legacy!

Vol. XXIII, No. 1, Spring 2012

LEGEND AND LEGACY IN NEVADA
DR. KENNETH MACLEAN

Robert M. Daugherty MD

- A tremendously interesting curmudgeon.
- He was very, very rude, abrupt, and abusive.
- He was one of my two physician heroes in Nevada.
- He wasn't in the business of medicine for money.
- Really a good doctor.
- He was the leader of the Board.
- The bme was run by the seat of the pants of Ken Maclean.

All of the above quotes from fellow physicians were describing Kenneth Frazer Maclean, physician who practiced surgery in Reno from1946 until his retirement in 1983. Ken Maclean, a native whose medical pedigree started with Joseph Lister, the father of antisepsis, included William J. Mayo, founder of the Mayo Clinic and ended with his grandfather, the first chairman of a department of surgery in the first university owned teaching hospital.

Ken was the leader of the Nevada Board of Medical Examiners for over thirty years. Thereby directly influencing the standards and quality of the practice of medicine in Nevada over three decades. It was during these three decades (1950-1980) that Nevada truly 'burst' on to the national scene going from a population of less than 200,000 to more than 1,000,000 people. It was without question, the dawn of a new medicine with technological and scientific advances beyond anyone's dreams when Dr. Maclean was appointed to the Board in 1949.

As the physician population increased from less than 1,000 in 1949 to over 4,000 in 1980, the board developed and established standards that determined the quality of medical care in Nevada into the 21st century. These newly established standards ranged from recognizing and licensing physician assistants to defining the criteria for legal abortion in the state, defining unprofessional conduct, establishing the process for investigating and penalizing physicians charged with violating the law, enumerating punitive action the board could impose on a physician found guilty of misconduct leading to a much more precise extensive document that served as the under pinning for the current Medical Practice Act.

Kenneth Frazer Maclean was born in Carson City March 9, 1914. His father, Donald Maclean, Jr., a graduate of the University of Michigan Medical School was the physician for the Nevada State Prison in Carson City. He later moved to the Riverside Hotel in Reno where the family lived, and his practice was located.

Kenneth graduated from Reno High School and the University of Nevada in Reno and received his medical degree from McGill University School of Medicine in 1939. World War II interrupted his surgical training at the University of Michigan in 1942. From 1942 until 1945, he served with the Univ. of Michigan Unit 298th General Hospital in the European Theater of Operations. Over twenty years later, Dr. Ken Turner, an obstetrician from Las Vegas was appointed to the Board.

Dr. Turner had been a private in the army as a glider and medical aid (army service preceded medical school) and had suffered serious injuries requiring several operations. Dr. Turner recalled that Dr. Maclean had been one of the first surgeons to operate on him after his evacuation from France to Liege Belgium where Dr. Maclean was stationed.

After the war, Ken Maclean continued the legacy of his grandfather and father by returning to the University of Michigan to complete his surgical training. At the completion of his training, He and his wife, Margaret, returned to Reno in 1947 to begin practice. Two years later, he was appointed by Governor Vail Pittman to serve on the Board of Medical Examiners.

The above description and accounts of Dr. Ken Maclean tell us a bit about the man, known as the czar of Nevada medical licensure for the over thirty years he served on the Nevada Board of Medical Examiners. He was considered a doctor's surgeon; a physician that other physicians would seek for their own personal surgical care.

But, if we stop and ask who was Dr. Ken Maclean and where did he come from? We find that he was the end of a legacy. It is a medical legacy that begins in Scotland with Joseph Lister and travels through the beginning of academic surgery in the Mayo Clinic.

Ken Maclean's grandfather, Donald Maclean, was born in Canada, received his medical education in Scotland and after serving in the Union Army during the Civil War; he became in 1872 the second chairman of the University of Michigan School of Medicine surgery department. He served as chairman for seventeen years. Included among his students was William J. Mayo, Mayo Clinic founder.

William Mayo graduated from the University of Michigan School of Medicine in 1883 and noted later in comments, "In 1882 Dr. Maclean began to practice asepsis and antisepsis while teaching about the work of Joseph Lister. In my first year I remember him being fastidious to operating room routine. Before surgery he would roll up his sleeves and carefully wash his hands before beginning an operation and again a couple of times during the operation." Dr. Mayo went on to say that one of the most important concepts he acquired as a student and assistant to Ken Maclean's grandfather was, "The sick man was the hub around which the entire education turned; the application of the art of medicine is based on the science of medicine." A concept that to this day, we admire and strive to instill in our students.

Thus, Ken Maclean brought a special legacy of medicine to Nevada. To better understand this legacy, we will go back and review the unique beginning of the Maclean family medicine legacy. Ken Maclean's grandfather became the chairman of the University of Michigan Department of surgery at the age of thirty-four in 1872. Donald Maclean, Sr., was born in Canada, educated in Edinburgh and received his medical degree and surgical training in Scotland.

After serving in the Union Army during the Civil War he moved to Michigan to practice. Apparently because of his success and popularity among his patients and students, he was appointed as professor and chair of surgery in Ann Arbor in 1872. At the time of his appointment, not only did the University of Michigan not have a teaching hospital, but neither did any other medical school in the United States. In fact, hospitals were not a part of medical care in this country until after the Civil War in the latter half of the 1880s. Individuals, who could afford medical care, would never be treated in a hospital. Hospitals as we know them today developed late in the 19th-century as scientific discoveries advanced medical care.

At the turn of the 19th-century, there were only two hospitals in the United States in Philadelphia and New York City. Massachusetts General became the third hospital in 1821. The first hospitals were originally established as infirmaries to provide for the poor, disabled and the infirm. For example, Philadelphia General, Bellevue and Baltimore General evolved from almshouses.

Thus, when the University of Michigan finished its hospital in 1877, there were fewer than two hundred hospitals in the country and none were university teaching hospitals. A remarkable legacy; Ken Maclean's grandfather, Donald Maclean was the chairman of surgery in the first university teaching hospital in the United States. However, his tenure ended abruptly in 1889 when he advocated the removal of the clinical of the medical school to Detroit against the opposition of both the board of regents and the president of the University. The regents instructed the president to request Dr. Maclean's resignation, which of course he did. In 1894, he was elected president of the ama. He died in Detroit in 1903 where he had moved in 1883.

We do not know how much Ken Maclean knew of his legacy? The fact that he chose to receive his surgical training at the place where his grandfather was the first chair would lead us to believe he did know of his grandfather. Unfortunately, he would not have known his grandfather who died eleven years before Ken was born. What we do know is that although the Maclean medical legacy ended with the death of Ken in 1985, the legacy does continue in Nevada through the standards of practice enabled by the actions of the Board of Medical Examiners under the leadership of Kenneth Maclean for over three decades.

Vol. XX, No. 1, Summer 2009

OUTSTANDING HOMEGROWN
DOCTORS OF NORTHERN NEVADA

John M. Davis MD

In the 1930s, there was a cadre of remarkable men native to northern Nevada, who entered into the study of medicine and returned home to become the foundation of the excellent medical community in Reno area during the last half of the twentieth century.

This group of men included Fred Anderson (surgeon and father of UNSOM), Donald Atcheson, Edwin Cantlon (surgeon and president of nsma, Vernon Cantlon (surgeon and president of nsma) (family practice), Arthur J. 'Bart' Hood (II), Dwight 'Dutch' Hood (internist and president of nsma), Louis Lombardi (surgeon and UN regent, Kenneth Maclean (surgeon and secretary of bme), and Leo Nannini (surgeon), Ernest Mack (neurosurgeon and chairman of wmc Trustees), Frank W. Samuels, obstetrics/

gynecology), (George Cann (internist), James Herz (founder of Reno Orthopedic Clinic, and William Arbonies (SMH radiologist).

These men attended the University of Nevada and came under the influence of Peter Frandsen, who stimulated their interest in science, guided them into medicine, and helped their admission to medical school. These schools included McGill, Michigan, St. Louis University, Harvard, Stanford, Cornell, Johns Hopkins, Northwestern, and Washington, St. Louis—some of the most prestigious institutions of the time.

It is quite remarkable and a tribute Professor Frandsen and the educational system at the University of Nevada that a small community fostered such an array of outstanding physicians. These men were instrumental in the development of Saint Mary's Hospital, Washoe Medical Center, and the ascension of medicine in northern Nevada. Their knowledge, skills, ethical standards, and influence served as a nucleus in attracting physicians with similar qualities to the area over subsequent decades.

Vol. XVIII, No. 3, Fall 2007

EDITORS' NOTE:

George Magee is a homegrown doctor, who was born in Yerington and practiced ophthalmology in Reno.

ELY COMMUNITY LEADER,
DR. WILLIAM BEE RIRIE

Lori Romero, Library Director of the White Pine County Library

Dr. William Bee Ririe was one of the most beloved citizens of Ely, Nevada. He was born in China on Christmas Eve, but he wasn't Chinese. He was the son of Canadian missionaries who were working deep in Western China. The name 'William Bee Ririe' will be well remembered in Ely, as the local hospital was named after him.

Dr. Ririe's first formal schooling was under the instruction of Quakers. He attended the American Quaker School in Chung King and later the China Island Mission School in Chefoo. He studied in 1913 at Oxford University in London, England, for a single year. He entered Toronto University in Canada, and he enlisted in the Canadian Army. During World War I he was sent to Europe and spent over two years on the Western Front as a medical corpsman.

When the armistice was signed, Ririe returned to Canada, and in 1918 he enrolled in an eight-year course of study in biological and medical sciences at Toronto University. He earned his MD in 1922. Dr. Ririe served an internship at hospitals in New York and Detroit. In October 1930, he accepted a position with the Nevada Consolidated Copper Company at their Steptoe Hospital. During the 'Great Depression' Dr. Ririe would accept any patient in need of medical care, even when he knew that his only payment would be a handshake.

In 1934, William Bee Ririe was married to Evelyn Dunn and transferred to Consolidated Copper's Hospital at Ruth, Nevada, but his devotion to the Steptoe Hospital kept him involved with the day-to-day operations there as well. During the fifteen years that he worked at Ruth and became an American citizen.

In 1949, Ririe transferred to Kennecott Copper Company's hospital in McGill, Nevada. After thirty-one years spent mending injuries and treating illness he retired from the company hospital in 1961. Purchasing a home across the street from the Steptoe Valley Hospital, he entered private practice of medicine.

When the copper company deeded the Steptoe Valley Hospital to the county, the younger doctors in town formed a new medical group, Eastern Nevada Medical Center.

In 1968, construction was begun on a new East Ely facility that opened in June 1969. By almost unanimous consent, the new hospital was named the William Bee Ririe Hospital. He continued to practice medicine, earning the honor of 'Physician of the Year' from nsma. The Nevada Industrial Commission also honored him for his contributions to the workingman. In March 1976, Dr. Ririe retired from practice. He died two months later.

Vol. VIII, No. 4, Winter 1997-98

SPUNKY KID
DR. GEORGE GARDNER

Roderick D. Sage MD

George M. Gardner must have been a spunky kid–bright and plenty spunky. He was born in Carson City January 30, 1875. His father, Matthew Gardner, was a Virginian who came west in 1803. He was a major landholder and lumber baron in the South Tahoe area (Gardner Peak was named in his honor.) As a youngster he played about his father's lumber mill and on the trains. About 1885 Matthew Gardner sold his lumber empire to E.J. "Lucky" Baldwin, the Nevada entrepreneur, and entered into the cattle business in Eagle and Smith Valleys.

George often helped his dad ship cows off to market. One day he lost his grip on the train coupling and fell under the wheels of a cattle car, crushing both his legs just below the knees. His legs went one way, and he went the other—in a wheelbarrow—to the nearest hospital. George survived, and perhaps it was at that time that he decided to become a medical doctor.

Deprived of his lower limbs at age twelve, and living in a relatively primitive area with little medical care, George was sent to live with an aunt in Oakland, California.

He attended a special school, where he prospered both intellectually and physically. With a working pair of cork legs and the determination to use them, he obtained an excellent high school education. George Gardner did well enough to gain admission to the first class of Stanford University, graduating four years later in 1895 in what has been described as 'that famous first class featuring among others, Herbert Hoover. Mr. Hoover worked his way through Stanford managing a laundry service. George often mentioned with some pride that his shirts and underwear were washed and ironed by a future president of the U.S.

Gardner entered Cooper Medical College in San Francisco, finishing the two-year curriculum in December 1896. Without the benefit of internship, this brand new twenty-two-year-old doctor signed on as physician and surgeon for a mining camp at Gold Creek, near Elko, Nevada, a move that had to take a lot of spunk. The following summer in 1897 he opened a medical office in Elko where he stayed until 1904, practicing in partnership with Drs. C.J. Hood and Samuel S. McDowell. In 1904, he moved again, this time to Fallon, Nevada.

During his early years in Fallon, Dr. Gardner contracted his services to the Newlands and Lahontan dam projects, the Fairview mining district southeast of Fallon, and the Tonopah Railroad Company. He also served the mining town of Rawhide, not only as a physician, but also as the town druggist. This arrangement ended when Rawhide burned to the ground with his apothecary shop.

For a while, Dr. Gardner owned a stage line serving Tonopah, Rawhide, Fallon, and parts in between. The stages were two big Royal Tourist cars, costing about $4,000 each. They held four passengers, and performed nobly, but service was often hampered by the fragility of their tires—George estimated that a tire would survive about fifty miles before a blowout. He spent $600 per year on tires alone. Dr. Gardner's pride and joy was a Pullman Touring car, which he purchased in 1911 for use in his busy practice in Fallon.

Because of his infirmity related to the leg prostheses, he engaged a number of young lads in Fallon to chauffeur him about on house calls (including this writer's father-in-law, Jack Price.) Dr. Gardner practiced widely in northern Nevada. He relates treating a miner in Carlin, Nevada, for a bullet wound in the hip, ultimately making twenty-three round trips by train to do so.

Other than his near fatal leg injuries, George's closest call came one Sunday morning when he stopped in a saloon for a glass of beer with a friend. A former patient, Joe Fuller, already in his cups, wrote him a check for $12 for an overdue fee then followed it up with a glancing blow to the jaw. This infuriated George, who immediately flattened the rascal with his cane. Fuller extracted a small pistol from his pocket. Fortunately it snagged briefly on the lining of his pocket, enabling George to make a fast exit. Fuller fired just as the saloon door slammed shut. In a panic, Fuller turned himself over to the county attorney, thinking that he had killed Dr. Gardner. He probably would have, too, but the bullet was deflected skyward by an iron brace on the barroom door, so much for Sunday fun.

Dr. Gardner remained in Fallon until 1917 when he removed his practice to Reno, joining Dr. Raymond St. Clair. In 1921 George's beloved wife, Louise, died during a major surgical procedure. After this George move to the San Francisco Bay area, opening an office in the Flood Building in San Francisco. He soon remarried, this time to Blanche Miller, a literate and charming former teacher. They made their home in the East Bay community of Kensington, which necessitated a daily commute by ferry to his office until 1937.

George sometimes removed his prostheses and stumped about on his foreshortened legs, reminding his friends of the famous French artist, Henri Toulouse-Lautrec. He practiced until 1946, when he retired so that he and Blanche could enjoy their elegant Lake Tahoe shorefront home near Meeks Bay during the summer months and his home in the Berkeley Hills in the winter months. George Gardner finally removed his cork legs for the last time and quietly died at the end of 1970, a month shy of his ninety-sixth birthday.

He was acclaimed to be one of the last surviving members of that illustrious first class at Stanford.

Vol. IX, No. 1, Spring 1998

EDITORS NOTE:

Raymond St. Clair was born in 1870 and attended Drake College. He received his MD from the College of Physicians and Surgeons in Keokuk, Iowa, in 1896. Licensed in Nevada in 1907 at Crippled Creek, he later moved to Reno, and was president of nsma in 1917.

FIFTY YEARS, ELKO COUNTRY DOCTOR
DR. LESLIE MOREN

Oral history by Owen C. Bolstad MD

Les came to Nevada in 1935 and helped to pioneer modern medicine in rural Nevada. Dr. Moren died quietly in his home in Elko on December 14, 1994, at the age of eighty. Les Moren was one of the founders of the Elko Clinic and was a driving force in the development of that group. A graduate of the University of Minnesota, Dr. Moren practiced medicine for over fifty years. He was active in civic affairs in his hometown and an avid supporter of organized medicine in Nevada. He served for many years as a delegate to the ama, and was elected as president of nsma in 1973. He served as a member of the State Board of Medical Examiners for over twenty years. Dr. Moren had been honored as 'Nevada Physician of the Year,' and as a 'Distinguished Nevadan.' His wife, Laurena McBride Moren, died in 1987. In 1992 working with the Oral History Program at the University of Nevada and with the support of the Great Basin History of Medicine Society, I had the privilege of doing a series of oral history interviews with Les. This culminated in the publication of a book entitled *Leslie A. Moren: Fifty years an Elko County Doctor.*

Perhaps some excerpts from the book would be the best memorial to this outstanding physician:

1937—"For a while I considered taking a residency . . . but I just didn't have the money. When I started practicing in Elko I got $200 a month and was surely glad to get that. In that era, none of the medical students that I ever spoke to went into medicine to make money. That was a secondary consideration. We all figured that we would have a comfortable living), but the idea of becoming a millionaire in the practice of medicine never crossed our minds. If you were a good investor and saved money you might, but you're not making it in medicine. I think that was a healthy attitude for us to grow up in. I think that may not be universally true today.

1946—(The Elko Clinic).... "We started talking partnership, because we thought that we could practice better medicine if we pooled our resources.... There were 4 of us—Dr. Robert Roantree, Dr. George Collett, Dr. Dale Hadfield and me. Drs. Charles Secor and A.J. Hood (Tom Hood's father) were made associates, since they were close to retirement age. We had our offices upstairs in what was the First National Bank building. You had to go up a two-tiered stairway.

1992—(Socialized medicine).... "Complete control of medicine by governmental agencies may occur in our country, as it has in other nations. If it does, I think that it will be devastating to many Americans, who will have to wait unconscionable lengths of time to have elective procedures done. You can't expect the physicians in a socialized system to work beyond the usual office hours when they will get their paychecks for just putting in the standard hours. I don't think that a government-controlled system is conducive to the practice of high quality medicine. Somebody said the other day that we would end up with a system that has the efficiency of the U.S. Postal Service. We may be in danger of developing a dual system, with proscribed government controlled medicine for the poor people and very expensive, high-quality medical care for the wealthy."

EDITORS' NOTE:

- That's the way Les Moren was–honest, open, and a square shooter. His friends, patients and organized medicine will miss him. There will never be another doctor quite like him.
- George Collett was born in Kansas in 1890 and graduated from Rush Medical College in 1922. He practiced in Crawfordsville, Indiana, before he moved to Elko in 1946. He briefly served on bme before he died in 1954. His son, Hugh, practiced in Elko.
- Dale Hadfield was born in Utah in 1916 and graduated from the Kentucky School of Medicine in 1942. In 1946, he was licensed in Elko, Nevada. He later moved to Tacoma, Washington.

- Robert Peter Roantree was born in Iowa in 1895. He received his MD from Washington University, St. Louis, in 1919. Dr. Roantree moved to Ely, Nevada, in 1920 and practice in Elko until he died in 1950. He was on the bme and president of nsma in 1931.
- Charles Edgar Secor was born in Michigan in 1882. He graduated from the Wisconsin College of Physicians and Surgeons in 1905 and was licensed in Cherry Creek, Nevada, in 1908. He moved to Tuscarora in 1914 and later moved to Elko. Secor was president of nsma in 1937.

Vol. VI, No. 1, Spring 1995

MOLLIE'S FOLLY
Doctors McKenzie, Hartzel, Krebs, and Maclean

Ryan Davis, History Student

In 1910, the Carson City News reported surgery by four prominent physicians, but current medical knowledge raises a doubt on their diagnosis. However, these doctors contributed to the advancement of Nevada medicine in the early 20th-century. On December 12, 1910, Drs. George McKenzie, Reine Hartzel, Ernest Krebs, and Donald Maclean, Jr., took part in the removal of sixty to seventy pounds of tissue from a prison inmate named Mollie Marrison [Harrison]. What was her diagnosis? Elephantiasis.

At first glance this event may not sound odd to the reader, but there are two glaring discrepancies in the medical report. "Well, for one, it is highly unlikely that a patient in 1910 could have over sixty pounds of tissue removed and survive," says Dr. John Iliescu, a retired Reno plastic surgeon. "The amount of fluid that would be lost by the patient alone would be enough to result in massive complications."

The other anomaly present is the diagnosis of elephantiasis. What makes the diagnosis odd is the area of the body in which it was diagnosed. According to Dr. Donald Maclean, Jr., who was the resident doctor at Humboldt State Prison and the man responsible for the diagnosis, "It was present in the woman's breasts."

Elephantiasis is a disease, primarily in the tropics, caused by filarial roundworms that inhabit lymph nodes, causing infection, inflammation, and swelling. This inflammatory swelling occurs mostly in the limbs of infected patients or in the scrotum of male patients. Since a female's lymph nodes that supply the breast are located primarily in the axillary region, it is highly unlikely that elephantiasis could ever occur in her breasts.

In light of these revelations, one must wonder what, indeed, was Molly Harrison's diagnosis. Was she the recipient of a radical, record breaking new procedure, or the victim of misdiagnosis?

It isn't as if the doctors who led the procedure were a group of mad scientists. Dr. McKenzie, the lead surgeon, was, in fact, one of the leading physicians not only in

Nevada but the entire West. Along with being one of the founders of Saint Mary's Hospital and its training school for nurses, he founded Mount Rose Hospital, which was a private hospital that existed for several years. He was president of nsma at 'the time the surgery took place, a member of the ama, and the American College of Surgeons.

He graduated from Rush Medical College in Chicago and after taking graduate courses at New York's Bellevue Hospital; he studied medicine at universities in London, Edinburgh, Glasgow, and Dublin. According to Sister Eulalia Cramsie who assisted Dr. McKenzie as a nurse at Saint Mary's, "McKenzie was an exceptional performer in those small, white-tiled surgical rooms. He was a fast worker at a time when total sterilization of the operating room was impossible. He was a wonderful surgeon."

Further research reveals no case of elephantiasis being diagnosed in a woman's breasts. Furthermore, no case of sixty to seventy pounds of tissue being successfully removed in any type of surgery was found in a review of 1910 medical journals.

Vol. XIV, No. 2, Summer 2003

EDITORS' NOTE:

Guy L. Rocha, Asst. Administrator for Nevada Archives and Records sent the following letter to the Editor: "I read with great interest the article entitled "The Mollie Folly" by Ryan Davis. I wanted to know more about this woman, so I looked for her prison inmate case file. Mollie was a black woman, age twenty-three in 1908, sentenced to ten years in prison in Carson City for second-degree murder in Winnemucca, Nevada. Her last name was Harrison not Marrison (a typo in the 1910 *Reno Evening Gazette* story) because the story in the *Carson City News* of December 11, 1910, has Harrison as Mollie's surname.

Dr. Donald McClean [Maclean] was the resident doctor at the State Prison in Carson City and not the Humboldt State Prison. In 1910, and for many years after, the only state prison facilities in Nevada were in Carson City. Dr. McClean [Maclean] mentions the operation in his report in 1910, which is part of the Prison Warden's biennial report in the Appendix to *Journals of Senate and Assembly* for 1911. In Harrison's prison record when she was seeking release from prison in 1911, she mentions the medical procedure and that she still has health problems despite the surgery. There is nothing more about the operation. It appears she was released from prison in 1913, as there are no records in her file after that date."

Further research by *Greasewood* staff reveals the following information. The surgeon was Dr. Donald Maclean., (1872-1938), the father of longtime Reno surgeon, Kenneth Maclean (1914-1985). The prison record indicates that Mollie "Killed a negro in her tent in Winnemucca with a knife." It further states under "marks, scars, moles, deformities, etc. Breasts abnormally large." She was paroled in July 1911 from her second-degree murder conviction.

NEVADA'S FIRST BLOOD TRANSFUSION

Dr. Vinton Muller

Dr. Vinton A. Muller writes in his brief biography about performing a blood transfusion, which he felt was the first ever done in Nevada. Dr. Muller, the son of a pioneer physician from Nevada City, California, and a 1917 graduate of the University of California Medical School had taken his surgical training under Dr. Wallace Terry.

Dr. Muller opened a surgical practice in Reno in 1920. Soon after he had arrived in Reno, Dr. Muller gave a paper on blood transfusion at a meeting of the Washoe County Medical Society. A short time later, he received a call from Dr. James Wiggins Gerow in Verdi, asking him to treat a woman who was critically ill after a post-partum hemorrhage.

Dr. Muller packed up his Kelley bottle set, some group II and group III typing serum (in those days blood was classified according to the Moss Classification), his microscope, hanging drop slides, and all the other equipment that might be needed. Rushing along in his Stutz automobile (one of two in the city of Reno) he drove to Verdi on the only road, which at that time was south of the Truckee River.

He typed the patient's blood and then tested 3 of her relatives before finding a suitable donor. Using a #6 needle on the patient and a #8 needles on the donor, he performed the transfusion, the entire procedure required from four to five hours.

EDITORS' NOTE:

Although various forms of transfusion had been attempted off-and-on for six hundred years. As late as the late 1800s, American physicians were experimenting with the use of cow's milk for transfusion and various other fluids.

It wasn't until Karl Landsteiner's discovery of the four major blood types (A, B, AB and O in 1901 that there was any reasonably scientific basis for transfusion of whole blood. For a time, the nomenclature devised by Jansky and Moss rivaled that of Landsteiner. Group I of Moss corresponded to AB, group II to A, group III to B, and group IV to O, so that it was really only necessary for Dr. Muller to keep 2 Moss sera on hand, groups II and III Landsteiner. Wiener did not discover the Rh factor until 1940.

Vol. I, No. #3, Fall 1990

LAS VEGAS' FORGOTTEN PHYSICIAN
DR. ROY MARTIN

Phillip I. Earl, Historian

Born at Table Rock, Nebraska, on November 16, 1878, Dr. Royce W. Martin was later to become one of Las Vegas' first physicians and the community's foremost booster. The son of a livestock buyer and dry goods merchant, he attended Wesleyan University for a year and received a business degree from Omaha Business College in 1898. For a time, he taught school in rural Nebraska before entering medical studies at University Medical College, Kansas City, Missouri, where he got his MD degree in 1903.

Known to his friends as Roy, he once told an interviewer that he had taken up medicine because of a boyhood experience. "I was born on a farm, and every time the doctor came, I got a dime for holding his horse. I decided then and there that doctors must have a lot of money and that was what I wanted to be."

Shortly after he graduated as a fledgling physician, he accepted a position with a mining company in Tampico, Mexico. Upon his arrival, he found himself in the midst of a yellow fever epidemic. Sent to a jungle district where one of the company's operations was located, he did his best to care for those down with the disease, who finally succumbed to the disease.

Following the subsiding of the siege, he returned to the United States. For a time, he practiced medicine in the northern section of the Oklahoma Territory on the so-called 'Oklahoma Strip' a section 28 miles wide and 100 miles long that had become America's premier 'outlaw country' by the turn of the century.

In July 1905, he heard of the boom in Goldfield, Nevada, and decided to try his luck as a doctor in Nevada. Arriving in Las Vegas by rail in August 1905 he learned that the community had neither a doctor nor a hospital, so decided to stay and set up a practice. He established an office in an 8'x10' frame shack near Fremont Street and was soon doing a booming business.

Four months after his arrival, he was appointed chief surgeon for the Las Vegas and Tonopah Railroad, serving in that capacity until the line ceased operations in 1918.

Mining was one of Dr. Martin's diversions over the years and he became a friend of every miner and mine promoter in southern Nevada, often accepting mining stock in exchange for his services.

Among the promotions he was involved in was the Three Kids Manganese Mine some fifteen miles southeast of Las Vegas, that boomed during World War I, and later became one of the nation's premier producers of strategic metal during World War II.

On June 27, 1910, Dr. Martin married Nellie Cotton at Seward, Nebraska. Not long after they arrived in Las Vegas, they moved into a new home on the corner of Fifth and Fremont Streets. By that time, he had moved his offices to the upper floor of the Thomas Building. He converted rooms to a hospital, one of Las Vegas' first, on North Second Street and was redoing the building for hospital when the Spanish Flu epidemic hit later in the fall. Dr. Martin was also Las Vegas' health officer at that time and not only treated patients, but enforced measures to close schools, theaters, churches, and saloons to check the spread of the disease.

On December 25, 1932, a new hospital opened in the 200 block of North Eighth Street.

Las Vegas had several physicians by that time and Dr. Martin had moved on. He served as president of the Las Vegas Chamber of Commerce for 10 years. He was also active with the Las Vegas Rotary Club, the Elks Lodge, the Masonic Order and the Eagles. He also worked on plans for the construction of Boulder Dam. In 1922, he was elected to the Nevada Assembly. He sponsoring legislation dealing with medical and dental practice in Nevada. He was concerned with highway legislation and taxation.

At the outbreak of World War II, Dr. Martin was retired and no longer practicing medicine, but the shortage of doctors at that time forced him to return to practice. In April 1943, officials at Basic Magnesium Inc. hired him to do physical examinations on prospective employees, and he and his wife moved to the Basic town site, Henderson.

In Nov. 1943 he suffered a series of heart attacks and died at Basic Hospital on December 22. He was survived by his wife and two daughters.

Although largely forgotten in Las Vegas today, Dr. Martin's imprint is on every aspect of the history of early Las Vegas. One of the city's middle schools was later named in his honor, but he deserves more recognition.

Vol. IX, No. 3, Fall 1998

EARLY DAYS IN LAS VEGAS AND RENO
DR. JOHN A. FULLER

Autobiography by John A. Fuller MD

Never will I forget my first impression of Nevada. I arrived on an evening train in the spring of 1910, after slogging it out in muddy roads and snow in a horse and buggy practice in a small Nebraska town for three years. As I got off the train in Las Vegas there was a full moon, and the desert seemed to pulsate with violet light glowing against the surrounding mountains. The air was pungent with the perfume of sage and greasewood, stirred up by a bunch of burrows, which was grazing nearby.

I was met by my future associate, Dr. Hal Hewetson—as picturesque looking a character as I have ever seen. He was dressed in khaki pants, which were stuffed into high leather boots, a woolen shirt and dirty sombrero, and a full beard. He had just returned from a prospecting trip in the mountains.

My new job was assistant railroad surgeon for the Los Angeles and Salt Lake Railway, and the main shops for the road were located here in Las Vegas. We had a small dispensary with four beds. There was no other hospital except a small private mine contract establishment kept by Dr. Roy Martin. We had no trained nurses—only male attendants trained by ourselves, no X-ray nor a laboratory—only test tubes and a few reagents. It was pretty primitive. We did not have a decent surgery. All of our major work we referred to Los Angeles, and we often accompanied the patient ourselves, hoping to keep him alive until we reached the 'City.'

Las Vegas in those days was a small town of between 1,500 and 2,000 persons. We had one school and two churches—a Protestant and a Catholic, one hotel—the 'Las Vegas,' and a large number of rooming houses over saloons. At that time there was a peculiar law that allowed only hotels to have bars. Naturally, the downstairs was occupied by the bar, with usually an outside stairway to the rooms above. There was only one main business street—Fremont—extending from the depot for five blocks and ending in the residential district. Standing on Fremont Street one could look down a side street, (Second Street, I believe) and view "Block Sixteen", a very prosperous Red light District. More on this later.

There were no paved roads in those days, only wagon trails. (Later, when I had acquired an automobile, it took me two days to drive to Los Angeles). Our medical practice was largely limited to Railroad men and their families. A trip out of town had to be made by train, although I made many a call by gasoline speeders, and even by railroad velocipedes if the distance were not too far!

I even delivered a woman on a train. I was called to the train to see a very sick passenger and found her in the last stages of labor. I could not take her off the train, as I had no place to put her. The only alternative was to get her into a 'stateroom' and with the help of passengers and the porter deliver her. Everything went off fine, except that the people never remembered to pay me, and it was thirty-six hours before I got home.

Speaking of our obstetrical practice, and there was plenty of it, as we had no hospital, it was necessary to deliver a woman in her own home. Usually we had a neighbor to help, but not always. We had no pre-natal care. Perhaps we would be engaged for such and such a time, but more often we were not consulted until the patient was in labor. If the patient lived some distance away, it meant 'camp' on the job until it was over, maybe all day. I recall one nerve-wracking case. I was called to see a patient in active labor and puerperal eclampsia. I had no help. Between Chloroform and Chloral hydrate, I delivered her by forceps, and both the mother and child recovered. Another case, and I had no help- this time, was one in which the delivery had been normal, I was attending the baby when I thought I heard a peculiar dripping sound. Turning to the mother 1 discovered the bed full of blood and she was hemorrhaging profusely. I will not mention my procedure, but I stopped the bleeding, and the woman made a slow but uneventful recovery. I mention these cases to show what the doctor had to contend with in those early days.

Automobiles were extremely scarce and I used a bicycle to get around. One time I had three cases of labor going at the same time. Remember, we had no hospital, so I was kept pretty busy pedaling from one house to another keeping track of their progress. I managed to confine two of the patients, but by the time I could get around to the third, I was greeted by a squalling new baby, and I was out ten dollars. That was the fee in those days.

At that time it was an unwritten law that a newly delivered woman remain flat on her back for nine days. I remember a healthy young woman whom I allowed to get up on the fourth day. She was so strong that I could see no reason for keeping her immobilized longer, but I thought for a while the old women were going to run me out of town!

Before I return to Reno, I want to refer back to a statement regarding the Red Light District. There were no more charitable and public minded people in town than the "girls down on the line." If a townsman were down on his luck, they were always ready to pass the hat to help him out. I was returning from Goodspring town about thirty-five miles away from Las Vegas, and I picked up a woman hitchhiker. I knew what she was, but this was desert courtesy. When we reached the edge of Vegas she insisted on getting out. She said it would hurt my reputation to be seen in her company.

While I was in Las Vegas, we had a real gold rush. Someone came in with a report of a rich strike in the mountains near the Colorado River. In no time at all, anything with wheels or four legs was commandeered. Everyone who could get away started out for the hills, some on foot. One woman, a waitress in the Railroad beanery was picked up about eight miles out in the desert, exhausted. She had no provisions, not even a canteen of water—an example of what hysteria could be caused by gold. The strike proved false, but there was plenty of excitement while it lasted.

And another example of mass hysteria: One day a prisoner in the local jail knocked out the jailer when he came in to feed the prisoners, and escaped. He was reported headed for the Colorado River. A large crowd started out after the man who was reputed to be a dangerous horse thief. The self-imposed posse was armed with everything from old shotguns to .22 caliber rifles. Fortunately none of them caught up with the fugitive. I do not recall if he were ever captured. The weather in Las Vegas used to get pretty warm in summer.

That was in the days before air-conditioning. I was called to Moapa one evening to attend some Railroad workers who had been overcome by the heat. When I arrived, I found one man dead and another still breathing faintly, although rigor mortis had already set in.

Although I was in general practice in Las Vegas, I came into contact with many eye injuries and infections, and it was through Dr. Hewetson's interest that I went east for a post-grad course. 1 cannot recall more than fifteen or twenty physicians in the community at that time. There were old Dr. Pickard, Dr. W.H. Hood, Dr. George McKenzie, Dr. Donald Maclean, Dr. Gerow, Dr. Sullivan, Dr. Bath, Dr. T.C. Harper, Dr. Horace Brown, Dr. William West, Dr. M.A. Robinson, Dr. J. LaRue Robinson, Dr. Morrison, Dr. George Servoss, Dr. St. Clair, Dr. and Dr. Parker Lewis.

Saint Mary's was across the street from the present hospital. The old Sister (I cannot recall her name) who had charge of the drug room, used to take the key to bed with her—

it was said—and if any supplies were needed during the night we had to wake her up.

The Washoe General at that time was only a county institution, it was a great deal later that it was enlarged and improved to accommodate private patients. We had no trained anesthetists. Anyone could pour ether. I recall one harrowing experience.

Most of these men were real characters. Dr. Pickard was said he never gave a bill to a patient. Dr. Hood was never to be seen without his pipe. I was told that he once carried it to the operative table. McKenzie was said to be the finest surgeon in the West. Dr. Bath gold-platted all of his instruments. Dr. Sullivan always wore a full beard. He would swear at a patient, and they enjoyed it. Once a patient, a small boy, had a redundant foreskin. I suggested he have a circumcision. He replied, "Oh Hell, let him wear it off." Dr. Horace was Exec. Sec. of NSMA when I was president.

When I moved to Reno in 1917, I associated with Dr. M.A. Brown. There were three small hospitals. Saint Mary's was the largest. Reno Hospital was operated by Dr. parker Lewis. Mt. Rose Hospital was a converted residence.

The patient was a rather husky man. The doctor himself went to sleep before the patient, who was just reaching the excitable stage. The patient suddenly rose up, jumped off of the table, knocked over the instrument stand, and nearly wrecked the surgery before he could be subdued.

Another time, Dr. Frank Samuels, Jr., who was really a very fine anesthetist, was working with me. The machine, a little old pump operated by an electric motor, caught on fire. With quick thinking Frank grabbed a sheet and threw it over the machine.

Some of our doctors can remember the annual Nevada State Medical Society meetings. We had some notable sessions at Elko, and at Ely when Dr. Bowdle was alive. But the real sessions were held in Reno, out at Bower's Mansion. We never lacked for essayists from the Bay region and Salt Lake City. Many of them came every year. Pop Gossi, of the Riverside Hotel, was the caterer. The day before the meeting he would go out to Bowers and build his barbecue pits, and we would have roast beef, Iamb, and pork. Being prohibition time, each member was assessed two pints. The only difficulty was to get an audience for the speaker. Most of the sessions were held around the improvised bar. Sometimes we had difficulty locating the essayist. I truly believe that we got more out of the informal discussions, and the old friendships rekindled, than from the most learned lectures of modern meetings.

In 1946, when I was president of the Nevada State Medical Association, we were just beginning to feel the pressure of Federal interference in medicine. I almost had to throw a government man out of my office one day who was insisting on making the State a Federal loan for Public Health, with the government, of course, telling us how to spend it.

During the First World War, a number of us old men were considered essential to the local medical needs.

We acted on the draft boards, giving a good half of our time without pay. The same conditions prevailed in the Second World War, but by that time we were deemed too old for service, so we served again on the draft board. The only recognition we ever received was a rubber-stamped signed certificate, thanking us for our services. We were not looking for reward or glory—we were only doing our part, as many others did who were unable to take part in actual combat, and we suffered the same deprivations of rationing. It was rather galling to call on the family of a 'civilian war worker' and find them sitting at the dinner table with a steak apiece.

Reno has progressed vastly from the time I describe. We have a fine modern medical center, with specialists that can be surpassed nowhere. Our hospitals have advanced enormously, with their modern laboratories and other conveniences.

As I look back to the old days, a feeling of nostalgia grips me, and I wonder if we were not actually happier under the old regime. They are all gone now, the old timers, and I guess I am the only one left—and I am expecting to read my obituary most any day!

To my son John, who was born in Las Vegas trip [illegible].

EDITORS' NOTE:

Dr. Joseph C. Elia preserved this typewritten monograph by Dr. Fuller and gave it to Dr. John Dooley, who permitted us to publish it.

"John Andre Fuller was born in Massachusetts in 1883 and received his premedical education in Omaha, Nebraska. He received his MD degree from the University of Nebraska in 1906 and interned at the State Hospital in Glenwood, Iowa. Licensed in Nevada in 1910, he practiced in Las Vegas from 1910 until 1917. At that time, he moved to Reno, where he practiced from 1917 until 1949. He died November 14, 1969. Ralph Bowdle was born in 1884 and received his MD from the Medical College of Ohio in 1909. He was licensed in Steptoe, Nevada in 1906 and president of nsma in 1921. Dr. Bowdle served on the bme."

Vol. XII, No. 1, Spring 2001

'MOST' ROMANTIC DOCTOR,
Dr. Washington Lincoln Kistler

Washington Lincoln Kistler, the youngest of thirteen children, was born in Pennsylvania in 1863. He developed an interest in medicine at an early age. At the age of eleven, he mastered the Morse code used by telegraphers, and in 1876 he became the youngest telegrapher employed by the Pennsylvania Reading Railroad, where he worked to earn money for his goal of going to medical school and becoming a doctor. Attending the University of Buffalo in New York, he graduated with a PhD in medicine in 1896.

He was planning to set up a medical practice in San Francisco when he booked passage on the Central Pacific Railway and headed west. The train stopped at the railroad division point in Wadsworth, Nevada, for fuel and water, and while he was stretching his legs on the station platform, he noticed the legs of a lovely young lady standing near the station. Dr. Kistler was smitten the moment he saw the young lady, and turning to his brother and traveling companion, he said, "That is the girl I am going to marry." After a short visit to San Francisco, he returned to Wadsworth, found the young lady, Pearl Patience Pike, set up a practice in Wadsworth, and after a whirlwind courtship, he married the girl in 1901.

Wadsworth at that time was a terminal for the Central Pacific Railroad, and Dr. Kistler was appointed as surgeon for the railroad. When the railroad moved its main terminal to Sparks, Nevada, the Kistler family moved there, where he continued to serve as railroad surgeon while he developed a general practice. The Kistlers had three children, two sons and a daughter.

In the early years of his practice the doctor used a horse and buggy to make house calls, then later used a Model T Ford to make his rounds. It is said that he was one of the founding doctors for Saint Mary's Hospital in Reno. While he was in general practice, Dr. Kistler developed a deep interest in the practice of anesthesiology and became quite adept at using ether anesthesia. He was often asked by other doctors to provide anesthesia during surgical operations. He died a premature death, reportedly from kidney failure due to ether exposure. In retrospect it seems much more likely that his that his early demise was the result of liver failure from chloroform exposure, an anesthetic agent known for its liver toxicity.

EDITORS' NOTE:

Reference: Dr. Kastler's granddaughter, Mrs. Gay Metcalf, who is associate librarian at unr Learning and Research Center, provided this material about Dr. Kistler.

Vol. XI, No. 4, Winter 2000-01

SOUTHERN NEVADA PIONEER DOCTOR
DR. JACK C. CHERRY

"Profiles in Medicine," *Nevada Health Review*, July 1981.

Dr. Jack Cherry most assuredly was a Nevada 'state treasure.' He came to us in 1924 after practicing in Montana for four years as physician for the Northern Pacific Railroad. That position gave 'Doc' many personal and professional awards, but the most prized was marrying his wife, Phyl.

"The mines were going strong in Goldfield, and I had done as much as I could do at Northern Pacific. I wanted to find a place of my own and get started," Doc remembers.

When he learned that Dr. Blake in Goldfield wanted to retire, Doc arranged to buy his practice and move to Nevada. Goldfield was lacking many niceties such as streets, sidewalks, trees, and grass.

Many of their friends and relatives couldn't understand why they wanted to go there. "But doctors were a dime a dozen then," said Doc. After they graduated they were all out looking for jobs, there was a depression during that time.

Thus, began a career that spanned more than fifty years administering to Nevada's citizens and helping to build our state's health care community. Even though the big companies were ending their mining operations when Dr. Cherry arrived in September 1924, the practice was extensive, and he began making a name for himself. "The big Goldfield Consolidated Mill was closed," Doc said. "Mark Bradshaw and Albert Silvers leased the tailings, which they washed down with hydraulic hose and treated with a cyanide process. They did so well that they refined the process."

"I had contracts with the three railroads, a mill, the mines, and Esmeralda County. My territory ran into Death Valley and as far south as Beatty." In addition he ran the Goldfield Hospital for nine years. Goldfield's closest call with an epidemic was a case of typhoid traced to the water supply. The water came from springs at Lida. It was pumped to redwood tanks, open on top, in a two-step process and then gravity fed into the town's wooden mains. The tanks were death traps for birds. Dr. Cherry said, "The tanks had to be drained and scrubbed down, but the privately owned water company didn't want the expense. It took a court order to get the job done."

"In those days most doctors didn't have a pot to sit on. My office in the Goldfield Hotel, two rooms on the second floor cost me $30 a month." There were quite a few bootleggers out in the hills at that time. Dr. Cherry recalls that some of them made real good corn liquor. The only other source was by prescription. He said, "The government allowed us 100 one-pint prescriptions every three months.

They were drawn on drug stores, and the empty prescription pad had to be returned to the irs in San Francisco. One of his regular customers was Walter Scott, 'Death Valley Scotty.'

He came to town regularly for his pint of bottled-in-bond. "He would arrive in a Model T Ford driven by an Indian," Dr. Cherry said. "He always wore a white cowboy hat, a white shirt, and a red necktie. For some reason he always rode facing backwards. Scotty constantly talked about building a castle. He was a big bullshitter.

His house was a 14' x 16' cabin in Grapevine Canyon." Scotty did get a castle, but in a roundabout way. He never had a dime to his name. It came about through an invitation to A.M. Johnson of Chicago to pay him a visit. Johnson had money, but not very good health. After a couple of months in Death Valley, he felt so much better that he decided to build a house. It became Scotty's Castle. Johnson kept more than one hundred men on the job, except during the scorching months of July and August. Dr. Cherry was the construction physician. "I'd drive the thirty-seven miles through Bonnie Claire and the Grapevine Mountains on Sunday, have dinner and conduct sick call."

Johnson wanted no shoddy monument He built it to endure. Cast iron sewer pipe coated with tar and wrapped with tarpaper. "I told him," said Dr. Cherry, "the pipe would last for fifty years in this dry climate, even without tar and paper." He replied, "I want it to last for 250 years." The castle's music room with its big organ reflects a special interest of Johnson. "He controlled the Wurlitzer business in Chicago," Dr. Cherry said. "The wrought iron fence and gate in the room were imported from a church in Spain."

Dr. Cherry moved to Tonopah in 1933 when Dr. Percy McCloud of that city died in a flaming car wreck while returning from Ely. On long trips across country the doctors carried extra gas, from five to fifteen gallons, in sealed cans. They made a funeral pyre. Cherry brought in Dr. Gerald Sylvain from Butte, Montana, to take over his Goldfield practice. Dr. Sylvain later moved to Las Vegas, where he still resides [1999]. Tonopah greatly expanded the territory Dr. Cherry covered, first in a Dodge, then later in a LaSalle coupe. He usually had a shovel strapped to the rear bumper. He administered to Round Mountain, Manhattan, Silver Peak, and Beatty. In Tonopah he took care of the 'Soiled Doves.' Every Monday the girls from the cribs arrived for their physicals. That night the police chief checked each for their certificate.

When World War II arrived, Dr. Cherry was offered a commission and went to the Presidio in San Francisco to talk with a general. "I cut

and it was high as hell." The result was a complete change of plans.'

I tried to stop the bleeding. "I took my blood pressure. It was high. Tonopah (elevation 6,000 feet) to Las Vegas (elevation 2,200 feet). Dr. Paul Jones, a hospital board member, invited him down to look over the town. His first check point was the National Hotel on Carson and 4th Street. Dr. Cherry settled into his new home fast. He took over the handling of county indigent cases, a responsibility that paid all of $400 a month. In the summer of 1942 he accepted the job of county hospital administrator when Paul O'Malley quit to run for justice of peace. That paid $650 a month.

The hospital was a small, struggling, overcrowded, somewhat makeshift institution with forty beds, patients often overflowing into the halls, a surgery lighted by spotlights strung along two pipes, a well for water and its own sanitation system—a septic tank. The city sewer didn't run that far out on West Charleston. It had two units, an old frame building with twenty beds used mainly for ambulatory patients and old folks, and a newer stucco structure with twenty beds. "When it rained we had to set out pans to catch the water in the old building," Dr. Cherry said. "We either had to have a new roof or a new hospital."

Since dependents of Nellis servicemen were treated there, further compounding the inadequacy of the facility, Dr. Cherry decided to use that as leverage to get federal funds to build a major addition. He went to Los Angeles to talk to officials of the Federal Works Agency. The initial sympathy of the Feds dissolved into silence. Apparently local opponents of the county hospital had got to them and blocked action. Dr. Cherry said, "For nine months nothing was accomplished. I couldn't even get a letter out of them. Finally, I called Pat McCarran." McCarran, then Nevada's senior senator, was surprised that the county was still awaiting word. "If that Los Angeles man doesn't call you in fifteen minutes, let me know," he told the Doctor.

The official's call was prompt, and typically mendacious. "We've been waiting for you," he said. "The plans are ready."

So the county got a $456,000 hospital addition by agreeing to come up with the $60,000 needed to equip it. That spawned a new problem. The linen demands for the additional 140 beds swamped the local laundries, so Dr. Cherry went through Los Angeles junkyards buying mangled washers, dryers, and a boiler. There was a headache with the railroad because ambulances carrying the sick and injured were frequently held up at the Charleston Avenue crossing. Dr. Cherry went after state and county funds to build an underpass. The new hospital was leased from the federal government for $1 a year, until such time as a bond issue could be floated to buy it. Through some tough bargaining, Dr. Cherry negotiated the Feds into accepting $182,000. And that is how Las Vegas got Southern Nevada Memorial Hospital.

The hospital is located on what was the county poor farm. In 1931, county patients were moved in and it became the Clark County Indigent Hospital. Ten years later a board was formed, private paying patients were accepted, and the name was changed to Clark County General Hospital with Dr. Cherry hired as administrator. During the early years in Las Vegas, Cherry was also physician for five of the Las Vegas hotels: the Flamingo, Sands, Riviera, Last Frontier, and El Rancho Vegas.

Jack Cherry has been state president of the Elks, Exalted Ruler twice, and was honored with a life membership in the Elks. His loyalty and love for Nevada strengthened through the years, and he was responsible for much of the growth and improvement in Las Vegas. During those years Dr. Cherry has known Nevada's people from grassroots miners and ranchers to the occupants of the State House. He knew the mountains, deserts, sagebrush, and cities. He gave Nevada the best that he had, and Nevada will remember him well. He died in 1986 at the age of eighty-eight.

Vol. X, No. 1, Spring 1999

WATCHFUL WAITING PHYSICIAN
DR. MORRIS WALKER

Autobiography by Dr. M.R. Walker

The unpaved streets were well dotted with saloons and gambling houses. There were uneven boardwalks in front of the businesses. Three railroads served the town, the Southern Pacific, the Virginia St Truckee, and a narrow gauge line serving northeastern

California points. There were several churches, several school buildings and a promising State University just north of town. Downtown there were three drug stores, an old opera house and three prospering banks. Only five or so doctors were actively practicing. There were no hospitals, so only emergency surgery was attempted.

It was the practice some fifty or sixty years ago, for medical colleges to send their graduates out to sink or swim with, generally, no intern training. The lives of the classroom, the clinic, and out in the world at large are quite different propositions. I received my diploma one afternoon about four o'clock. I had already bought my medical and surgical cases; also a few textbooks. I took the train for Reno at 7 p.m. knowing full well that I was ill prepared for the work, responsibilities and the uncertainties of the near future. However. I went with a determination to make good; I must survive or perish; I no longer would have a friendly professor to advise me.

I was not long getting settled in my office. It was a tiresome and discouraging experience, waiting, waiting, for the sadly needed patients. Finally one evening about five o'clock a call came from an old Englishman (a druggist). There had been a runaway, a girl was thrown out of the cart, was badly hurt. Would I come at once? I grabbed my medicine case and ran. I found the young woman unconscious but could find no outward marks of serious injury. The young woman was taken to the nearby home of a relative for the night. I proceeded to put on an appearance of professional seriousness and to do "watchful waiting," at the same time keeping relatives and friends doing all sorts of errands.

Towards morning the girl revived and before night left for her own home. The "strange doctor" became the subject of comments and inquiries. (Advertising?) I received profuse thanks from the family. No cash. However, the ice was broken. The family later on gave me many calls—and some cash.

Late one afternoon, a week later, a row and robbery took place in one of the many saloons. The chief of police (he constituted the entire police force) was called. The robber made a break, and ran into the willow thicket that lined the riverbank. Shots were exchanged. The chief was shot through the lower abdomen. As usual on such occasions, all the known doctors were called. While everyone was engaged with this affair one of the older doctors, Doctor Gibson, received an urgent call to go out to the mines some five or six miles from town. As he was busy he called the new man (myself) to make the call for him.

I had not as yet bought a horse. I borrowed a bicycle and struck out for the mines. I found a woman desperately ill with pneumonia. She was living in a miner's shack. I gave emergency treatment and returned to report to Dr. Gibson, who promptly turned the case over to me, as he had no time to attend the patient. (Later I learned that it was a charity case).

I, of course, was eager to take over. I found a kindly neighbor, who was also a graduate nurse, to take over the nursing and on the side look after the woman's five little children. I stuck around counting out a few tablets, giving many orders, trying to look wise and professional. The nurse, with consummate skill, brought the woman through to recovery. There is an interesting history connected with this patient. Her husband was a miner. About a week before, he had been killed in a mine accident, leaving his family all but destitute. The death and the widow's sickness aroused the sympathies of the entire camp.

Some six months earlier John Sparks, then Governor of Nevada, purchased the mine. He and his wife were noted for their charities and neighborly acts. Mrs. Sparks visited the sick woman, often bringing substantial aid. Mrs. Sparks asked me to spare no effort or expense and to keep her informed as to the progress of the disease. Some four or five weeks later she handed me two twenty-dollar gold pieces as her contribution. As the patient did recover, the new doctor was given a "great hand." His fame spread.

EDITORS' NOTE:

Reference: An autobiography written by Dr. M. Rollin Walker published in 1945, *A Life's Review and Notes on the Development of Medicine in Nevada*. After graduating from the College of Physicians in San Francisco in 1901, Dr. M. Rollin Walker immediately moved to Reno, Nevada, and located his practice there. Reno at that time was a bustling Western town of 4,000. Dr. Walker is truly one of Nevada's most significant medical historians.

Vol. II, No. 3, Fall 1991

DUELING PHYSICIAN
Dr. Kurt Hartoch

Dr. Hartoch's Oral History by Linda Dufurrena

Kurt Leopold Hartoch was born in Dusseldorf, in the Republic of Germany on June 7, 1908. Son of a middle-class merchant, he suffered during the post-World War I famine and inflationary period. While studying at the university, Hartoch became a member of a dueling society. At German universities dueling societies occupy a niche that may be likened to Greek fraternities on campuses today. Although the stated objectives of the dueling societies were to promote physical exercise, discipline and swordsmanship, the most sought after goal was a handsome dueling scar upon the graduate's face, preferably on a cheek, as a symbol of one's status. Kurt Hartoch proudly displayed his dueling saber on a wall in his home and the dueling scar across his nose.

Dr. Hartoch was a unique person with a fine German medical education. He could have practiced anywhere in the world, but circumstances and choice led him to practice in a small rural community in western Nevada. He was educated at the University of Köln (Cologne)/Rhine at a time when German medicine was rated among the best in the world. In early 20th-century, American doctors traveled to Europe for training. Germans were leaders in medical research.

Although Kurt Hartoch became a naturalized American citizen in 1935, he never really lost his rich guttural way of speaking and his brusque Teutonic mannerisms. His family wanted him to become an attorney, and he did study law for a period of time at the University of Köln, but found the subject boring and switched to medicine. He was proud of his German medical education, which at that time was quite different from our American system. German students read medicine under the guidance of a professor, employing a loose curriculum. The success or failure of a student depended entirely upon the diligence of the student and his success was not known until he completed one final comprehensive examination lasting for six months.

Kurt scoffed at the tightly controlled American system, feeling that the educators 'spoon-fed' their students.

With the encouragement of his farsighted parents, the new Doctor Hartoch left Germany soon after graduation. He immigrated to Los Angeles, California. There, he obtained an unpaid position as an extern at the Cedars of Lebanon Hospital, working there for about 6 months. In November 1935 he traveled with a friend to Carson City, Nevada, to appear before the State Board of Medical Examiners to obtain his Nevada medical license. During the journey to Carson City, they encountered ice and snow, skidded off the road, and rolled down a steep embankment. Kurt suffered two broken ribs. Returning to Cedars of Lebanon Hospital, he was promoted to the exalted rank of intern, with room and board as well as $10 salary per month. During his time as an intern at Cedars, he had the opportunity to examine and treat a number of Hollywood notables, including: Al Jolson, Ruby Keeler, Alice Fay, Charlie Ruggles, and Arthur Treacher. This interesting internship ended in July 1937.

Opening his practice in the Cheney Building on South Virginia Street in Reno in 1937, he struggled alone against the established medical groups in the community. Living in an apartment, he cooked his own meals, washed and ironed his own clothes, and scrimped to save his meager supply of money. Washoe County Physician, Dr. George Cann, guessing Dr. Hartoch's rather dire straits, appointed him Assistant County Physician—a post that paid a princely $50 per month. While serving in this position, Dr. Hartoch achieved a brief moment of national fame one winter when he traveled with a driver and guide in a homemade snowmobile into the high country near Weber Lake in the Sierra Nevada Mountains to minister to a suffering caretaker at Hobart Mills. They struggled through snow and ice for fifteen hours, leaving the good Samaritan tired, hungry and aching all over from the bumpy ride.

As a county physician it was his duty to attend indigent expectant mothers, and since transportation was not available.

He was also expected to make regular prenatal visits and deliver babies at home. On one occasion he delivered a premature infant weighing just over one pound in a home in Washoe City. The little tyke was put into the proverbial shoebox lined with cotton and got along just fine. While practicing in Reno Dr. Hartoch was approached by a number of representatives from Winnemucca, who urged him to move to their community. When the boss of the Getchell Mining Company promised to send their industrial cases to him, Dr. Hartoch decided to check out the town. The first visit to Winnemucca was not promising (at that time the entire state of Nevada had a population of something over 100,000). A second visit was encouraging, and after due consideration, the decision was made to move to Winnemucca.

His first office consisted of four upstairs rooms accessible only by a steep 'neck-breaking' staircase, with the rooms divided by board partitions. There was no insulation, and the place was heated by single oil stove. After ten years, Dr. Hartoch moved his office into an old bakery building next to the post office on Fourth Street, spending about $7,000 to convert the space into a medical office. It was not until 1962 that he built his own modern and well-designed medical office building on the corner of 5th and Bridge Streets in Winnemucca.

When Hartoch first arrived in town, the hospital was old and inadequate, with long dark corridors. It was run by a single nurse, Wilkie Pinson. She was the head nurse, receptionist, bookkeeper, x-ray technician, laboratory technician and bill collector. She was the medical authority for the city and county, and really ruled the roost.

After the move to Winnemucca, Dr. Hartoch's wife remained in Reno until they sold the property that they owned. In Winnemucca they lived in a house on Garrison St. where in January 1942 daughter Carole was born. In August 1943, Mrs. Julia Hartoch underwent a minor surgical procedure at Saint Mary's Hospital in Reno. Something went awry during the operation and within a month she died from complications of surgery.

In 1948, Kurt married Wilma Peraldo. They had two children: a son Mark, who was killed in a truck accident in 1987, and a daughter, Marlese, who is now living in California.

In the 1940s, the cost of medical care was low. Dr. Hartoch' s fee for an office visit was $2 or $3, depending upon the severity of the patient's problem. A hospital visit was more expensive, as was a house call–$5. He made house calls until he closed his practice in 1983. Prenatal care, delivery and postnatal care was $150, but during WWII he delivered many babies for a total charge of $45 because that was what the government would pay.

From time to time, Dr. Hartoch dabbled in business investments, not all of them successful. In 1939, he was offered some mining property for $100 (5¢ a share.) He refused this offer and was chagrined a few years later when a mining company bought up those shares for $16.40 per share. Then, he became involved in mining on Willow Creek, buying a number of claims and grubstaking a miner to work the claim. When he caught the miner selling off the gold nuggets produced in the mine, that enterprise suddenly folded. He bought stock in Bullion-Monarch Mining Company, selling it when the stock went up. Later the same company asked him to reinvest, which he refused to do. This property developed into one of the largest gold producers in the United States. In 1950, he grubstaked a prospector who wanted to mine the riverbed of the American River, but that enterprise fell apart. He invested in a mining venture in the Rochester District, but that didn't turn out well either.

His practice was a well-balanced mixture of general medicine, surgery, obstetrics and industrial medicine. He thought that he had delivered more than 2,000 babies during his career. On many occasions he was asked to make country calls, sometimes as far away as the Oregon border. He made many calls to the scenes of accidents in mines, ranches, and train wrecks. He cared for black families and Mexican families. He cared for prostitutes and itinerants. He cared for Indian families and had a special place in his heart for them.

With a wide and varied practice, he had many devoted patients and maintained a fine reputation in his chosen community.

In 1983, at the age of seventy-five, Dr. Kurt Hartoch retired from the practice of medicine. Health problems began to take their toll. He became almost blind due to uncontrollable glaucoma. He continued to enjoy life with his beloved wife, Wilma, surrounded by his collection of art, stamps and coins. He enjoyed visits with his two daughters, Carole and Marlese, both living in southern California.

EDITORS' NOTE:

Dr. Kurt Hartoch died in Winnemucca, Nevada, September 19, 1995, at the age of seventy-eight from the infirmities of age. His passing was memorialized by his daughter, Carole Flaxman, who endowed a gift of $1,000 to the Great Basin History of Medicine Program in memory of her father. Some material in this article was taken from a series of oral history interviews done in 1993 by Linda Dufurrena who is a Humboldt County historian, photographer, and a former patient of Dr. Hartoch.

Vol. VI, No. 4, Winter 1995-6

AMERICA'S PATHOLOGY LEADER
DR. JIM BARGER

Oral history by Lisa Puleo, Clark County Medical Society

I, Jim Barger, was born in Bismarck, North Dakota, at Saint Alexis Hospital. My father was a country banker and my mother, a native of Wisconsin, was a homemaker. I had an older brother, whose name was Thomas. Our parents, who were 'good' Irish-Catholics, wanted one of us to become a priest. I went to school in Linton, North Dakota, graduating from high school in 1934. After spending two years at Saint Mary's College in northern Minnesota (now St. Mary's University) I transferred to the University of North Dakota.

My brother was supposed to enroll in premed, but after he had been there for a week he transferred to mining engineering.

He also joined the Kappa Sigma Fraternity, although our parents did not approve. I wanted to become a chemical engineer, but mother asked me, "Why don't you try premed?" Well, one cannot "just try it" and once I was in premed, I was caught.

After graduating from medical school, World War II came along. I was sent to Fitzsimmons Army Hospital in Denver, Colorado. This was during the early days of blood transfusion. I gave a paper on alkaline phosphatase in Portugal, and while there I met Phillip Levine, a pioneer in blood banking. He stimulated my interest in the Rh system, so when I returned to Fitzsimmons I began to do some research. Phil Levine and others were making anti-Rh serum by injecting rhesus monkey blood into Guinea pigs. When I tried to do that, I ran into the problem of obtaining rhesus monkey blood.

The tuberculosis hospital in Denver was run by a church group, which had a monkey colony. I went over and looked at their monkeys, and they were almost as big as me—boy, were they tough! I decided that I couldn't handle that job, so I went over to the Zoo and asked for help. The zookeeper very nicely got me the rhesus monkey blood. When I got back to Fitzsimmons, I ran into the chief of service, a colonel, who asked me, "Where have you been?" I replied, "To the Zoo, Sir," and he said, "What for?" I told him, "To get some rhesus monkey blood, Sir," and he asked, "What for?" I told him that I was trying to make some Rh anti-serum. He looked at me, smiled and just walked away. I didn't get Guinea pigs to make the antiserum, and soon received orders to leave Denver.

I was transferred to the General Dispensary in Washington DC. The dispensary opened in January 1943. It was great at the dispensary—we wouldn't look twice at anybody in the clinic unless they had at least three stars. I stayed there until 1944 when I was transferred to the Office of American Affairs. They sent me to a hospital in a jungle town in Eastern Bolivia. At the hospital I met Sister Mercy. I spent fourteen months there, traveling to nearly every place in eastern Bolivia.

I was looking for beriberi that had been reported in that region in 1915 or 1920. By the time I got there, beriberi had been practically eradicated. When I searched for patients with beriberi, I was always told that they were a little bit further into the interior. I finally got to a place that was in the middle of the Amazon jungle, when I decided that beriberi could just stay there.

I married Susie right after I came back from Bolivia. We were married in Douglas, Arizona. I was sent to Colorado Springs, Colorado, but by that time, I was on my way out of the service. Susie and I had two children, James Jr. (who will be fifty this year) and daughter Susan Mary. My wife, Susie, died in 1951. I later married my second wife, Josephine. She developed carcinoma of the lower esophagus and stomach. She died from disseminated intravascular coagulation. My third wife, Janie, died from emphysema secondary to smoking. She was always trying to quit, but finally just didn't have any lungs left. After she died I would find packs of cigarettes hidden here and there in the house. She was a typical addict and was always trying to hide her habit.

I came to Las Vegas from Phoenix, Arizona, in 1964. I got a job at Sunrise Hospital with a pathologist I knew when I was in Phoenix. It was a nice place to work because I could do what I wanted. The administrator, Nate Adelson, was one of the toughest negotiators I have ever known. When you reached an agreement and shook hands on it that was it. If he made a mistake he ate it, and if you made a mistake, you ate it. He was fair, but tough, and he was a great guy. He was the one who built Sunrise Hospital. There were other pathologists in Las Vegas when I arrived. [Bob] Belliveau and [John] Grayson were at the County Hospital, and my group was at Sunrise. There was enough work to keep busy, and so it was nice.

About that time I started getting involved in the national politics of medicine and pathology. When I first arrived in Las Vegas, it was a small, growing town, with not a very big medical group. I knew everyone. We had frequent meetings, and it congenial— a thing that I now miss.

We would get together and get to know each other. I think that kind of comradeship leads to consultations and exchanges of ideas.

I have always been a member of the medical society, no matter where I was. If you are going to be a physician, you should be a member of the ama. Most of the doctors in town were members of the ama. Everybody seemed more relaxed in those days. I think we should go back to having county society meetings where we could just get together and become better acquainted. We used to have a pathology society too. We would meet about once every three months and have dinner. I was selected as a delegate to the ama by the county medical society. We had great times at the ama and the county meetings. It was fun in those days, and I wish we could bring those days back. I think people are too busy these days. As the saying goes, "Take a real interest as though it all really mattered!"

EDITORS' NOTE:

This story is an excerpt from an Oral History done by Lisa Puleo, executive director of the Clark County Medical Society. Dr. Barger was president of The College of American Pathologists 1981 to 1983.

Vol. X, No. 4, winter 1999-2000

DR. STAHR MAKES A HOUSE CALL

Roderick Sage MD

Dr. Roland Stahr was a revered pediatrician in Reno from 1939 until his untimely death in 1969, and before that in Fort Dodge, Iowa, where he had practiced for the previous dozen years. He was a hero, not only to his young patients and their parents but to his colleagues as well, serving as president of the wcms and nsma. He was named Nevada's Outstanding Physician in 1965.

In 1937, Roland Stahr practiced in Fort Dodge, a city of 20,000 inhabitants in northern Iowa. He was a consultant to doctors all over that part of the state for general childcare and also for pediatric allergies.

My father was such a general practitioner in the nearby town of Eagle Grove, twenty-five miles to the northeast. He often referred his difficult pediatric problems to Dr. Stahr. The onset of such a request would begin with a terse phone call, "Stahr? This is Sage."

In the summer of 1937 Iowa endured an epidemic of poliomyelitis, then generally known as infantile paralysis. One morning in mid-July, when my father and mother were enjoying a two-day visit with friends in Des Moines, I awoke to an overwhelming sense of lassitude. After nearly falling asleep in my morning cereal, I tumbled back into bed with covers drawn up and window shades down. Thus I remained, cocoon like, all day until the folks returned in the late afternoon. They wondered if we shouldn't cancel a planned trip to visit relatives in Waterloo—one hundred miles to the east. However, the next day I awoke bright eyed and bushy tailed, 'rarin' to go. We had a splendid 'two-day get-together.'

The day after we returned home, whatever it was, hit the fan! In addition to a return of that overwhelming weariness and photophobia, there was also a crushing headache, fever, and a steamroller overall aching. "I wasn't just under the weather, I was sick." Then the fun began.

"Stahr? This is Sage." After a few hours of observation and a downhill course, another call and Roland Stahr was on the scene—the first of 3 house visits he made from Ft. Dodge that night.

The physical exam was an ordeal. A few days before I had been a lively, nimble eleven-year-old swimming in the town pool, playing softball, and 'rassling' with my older brother. Now sitting up in the bed was a chore. Groaning with misery I braced myself with my arms. It hurt to extend my legs more than 60 degrees. The flashlight hurt my eyes and my neck was sore and inflexible. Would that examination ever end?

After a while (after it was dark) Roland returned, armed with paraphernalia. "Okay, Roddy, we're going to have to get blood out of your arm."

Ouch! But it was over in a hurry. Then, the big surprise. "Okay Roddy, lie over on your side. We're going to put a needle in your back so that we can draw out some fluid."

Over on the left side, knees drawn up, and back convex. This effort hurt, and I grunted and perspired. The stick in the back was accompanied by an odd, deep nerve aching. In a bit this ordeal ended, lights went out and I was able to get some sleep. But believe it or not—it must have been 2:00 AM—here was this gadfly and his companion, my father, back to torment me some more.

This time they arrived with an enormous vial of watery-looking fluid, a giant syringe and a long, skinny needle. The neurological exam was repeated. I was aware of more pain and increasing weakness. This had become a true pediatric emergency. Into the arm vein went the contents of the vial by way of the big and long needle. This seemed to continue for an eon, until the needle finally came out. Tape and cotton were applied to the arm and at last I was in dreamland again. The remainder of the night was one of blissful slumber.

On 'coming to' at 8:30 AM the whole world was bright and rosy. Fever down, stiffness and aching nearly gone, my spirits were hearty. To recapitulate a bit: As I lay there in my misery, I heard those two men, Dr. Roland Stahr and my dad, Dr. Erwin Sage talking about me. The word "polio" was bandied about. That didn't sound too ominous. Dr. Stahr said something about a positive Babinski sign, so it couldn't be anything bad. Then he told dad that he had had two patients with this unknown malady polio who received the same sort of serum; one did very well, but the other didn't.

That July afternoon and evening, when it became obvious that I was one sick cookie, the big wheels started to turn. Roland Stahr arrived on the scene and checked me out. He went out and returned later with his diagnostic kit to draw blood and do a spinal tap. The disease was moving fast! When the diagnosis of polio became evident, father called the state health department in Des Moines, eighty miles away and ordered a batch of poliomyelitis convalescent serum.

This was how the disease was treated in its early phase in 1937. Venous blood, drawn from recovered polio a victim was spun down, leaving clear serum loaded with anti-polio antibodies. This serum was injected into the patient's vein. Later it was found that most people had the antibodies, probably from subclinical infection and the serum was more widely obtained.

At midnight father was on his way to Ames, Iowa, to rendezvous with a state trooper who had transported the precious supply of serum from Des Moines. By 2:00 AM he was back home, and Dr. Stahr was once again on hand to do the honors.

The first batch worked for five days, giving way to a relapse with more fever, headache, muscle pain and weakness, but this time a new supply of serum was obtained under less hectic conditions. After this injection I was home free.

Later when I asked my dad the name of my illness he replied, 'anterior poliomyelitis.' Big deal. Then I asked him what that meant in ordinary language. He answered, 'infantile paralysis.' In 1937, those two words engendered terror in the beholder. For a moment I was scared out of my wits, and asked him if I was going to be paralyzed. He assured me that I wasn't, but let me know that I had luckily missed that fate.

Roland Stahr came west to Reno in 1939, after suffering a debilitating problem with arthritis, which persisted for years until he was serendipitously tested for Bang's Disease (brucellosis). He reported that the ensuing orchitis clinched the diagnosis and he was then successfully treated for chronic brucellosis.

When I started my dermatology practice in 1958, Dr. Stahr was on hand to welcome me and introduce my wife, Jackie, and me to the community. He was a superb consultant for a fledgling dermatologist, and is still a hero to the four young Sage brothers.

Vol. IX, No. 3, Fall 1998

DOCTOR ON IWO JIMA (WORLD WAR II)
Dr. Robert Locke

Dr. Bob Locke was a quiet, modest man, who did not brag about or mention his bravery during World War II. Although it was known that he had been awarded the Navy Cross, his account of privation with honor on Iwo Jima was found after his death. He never forgot his university and served as a full-time physician at the student health facilities.

Bob was born in Mt. Pleasant, Utah, in 1920. The family moved to Reno 10 years later. When he attended the University of Nevada, he came under the influence of famed Professor Peter Frandsen, who was responsible for many Nevada students pursuing careers in medicine and dentistry. While Bob was attending the University of McGill Medical School in Montreal, Japan bombed Pearl Harbor. The following year, Bob enlisted in the u.s. Navy, and in 1943 after graduation, Ensign Locke reported for active duty at Treasure Island in the San Francisco Bay. He volunteered for Marine Corps duty, but further training was interrupted by the desperate situation in the Pacific.

Hurry-up exercises on Maui's beaches did not prepare Battalion Surgeon Locke for the horror that was to follow on Iwo Jima. He wrote, "Intensive education as to the exact landing location occupied the last two weeks prior to landing, along with ddt dusting and wax impregnation of all combat clothing to prevent typhus and other pest-borne disease." Then, what history would record as one of the bloodiest battles of the Pacific ensued. The Japanese deliberately ignored the first wave of U.S. troops on the beach of Iwo Jima in order to trap them and the second wave on the narrow strip of sand.

Senior Officer Locke was placed in charge of the second wave of vehicles on the right flank, but as his lead vehicle reached its goal, "The radio fairly screamed us back to sea in that we were definitely in Japanese territory." As they regrouped, intense mortar fire erupted destroying all landing craft and pinning them down on thirty feet of beach.

During the intense enemy fire, Locke remembered, "I made a flying leap off the front of the vehicle and landed in neck high water and waded on in to my unit." A few seconds later his vehicle and the remaining occupants were annihilated. "For the next seventy-two hours we were totally confined to the narrow beach strip." Locke's Navy Cross citations read, "An adjacent unit was in the center of the heaviest concentration of artillery and mortar fire and was suffering extreme casualties beyond the abilities of its depleted medical sections. With total disregard for his own safety, Lt. J.G. Locke voluntarily left his covered position and entered the shelled area four times and helped carry wounded to the evacuation station." Locke: "almost every foxhole that I visited blew up within seconds of my leaving."

During the following twenty-one days, the Japanese continually killed Americans by creeping out of the tunnels at night and infiltrating their positions. Locke, "It was discovered that the Japanese were infiltrating in American uniforms during the night in small groups and were swimming to sea and coming back in on the beach."

The second part of Locke's citation notes that under enemy fire Lt. J.G. Locke waded out to a small boat evacuating the wounded and forced the crew that refused to leave because of the intense fire to take the wounded off the island. At the end of the Iwo battle Dr. Locke wrote, "Actually, the flag raising on Iwo was very premature to those of us there and was far from the climax. Probably the true climax was our cemetery trips, the last few days before final securing of the island, through the thousands of dead lined beside rows of crosses, attempting to identify and locate lost friends."

After Dr. Locke returned to Reno, he was appointed to the wmc medical staff on July 2, 1947. In 1951, Washoe Trustees agreed with the medical staff's recommendation that he manage all patients on the tuberculosis ward. He practiced internal medicine for thirty years. Dr. Locke died at eighty-two.

Vol. XIV, No. 1, Spring 2003

DOCTOR IN FRANCE (WORLD WAR I)
DR. ALICE THOMPSON,
NEVADA'S FIRST FEMALE PATHOLOGIST

Anton P. Sohn MD

No physician in Reno's history had more blue blood than Alice Lillian Thompson, who is the granddaughter of Myron C. Lake of Lake's Crossing fame and the acknowledged founder of Reno. Alice born January 4, 1876, on the Lake Ranch south of Reno attended the Normal School (Teachers College) of the University of Nevada graduating in 1897, and taught school for fourteen years before attending the Oakland School of Medicine. She transferred to the College of Physicians and Surgeons, an eclectic medical school in San Francisco, and graduated in 1914 specializing in pathology and laboratory technology. Dr. Thompson interned at the San Francisco City and County Hospital before leaving the Bay Area to become laboratory chief of Santa Barbara Cottage Hospital. True to the American patriotic spirit, she joined the war effort during wwi and directed the laboratory at Base Hospital Unit No. 47 in Beaune, France.

After the war, Dr. Thompson returned to Nevada and became its first known female pathologist. She was licensed in Reno in 1920 and became director of Saint Mary's Hospital Laboratory and the State Hygienic Laboratory—now the Nevada State Public Health Laboratory. In 1934 Dr. Thompson became the first full-time pathologist at the Washoe County Hospital (now Renown Regional Medical Center) with a salary of $200 a month. That same year, the Board of Trustees authorized the hospital to refer all of its laboratory tests to the State Hygienic Laboratory for $50 a month.

During WWII Dr. Thompson was physician for the Reno School System. She also was physician for women at the Univ. of Nevada for over twenty years. She died December 3, 1960, at 84.

EDITORS' NOTE:

References: *Reno Evening Gazette*, December 3, 1960, "Dr. Alice Thompson Pioneer Doctor Dies."

Vol. XXII, No. 1, Spring 2011

CHAPTER IX:
THE HOOD DYNASTY
DOCTORS HOOD HISTORY OF MEDICINE LIBRARY

The Doctors Hood History of Medicine Library, located in the Savitt Library at the School of Medicine, is named to honor the Doctors Hoods, who have practiced medicine in Nevada since 1886 when Dr. William Henry Hood settled in Battle Mountain until 2002. Five of his relatives have also practiced in our state. These include William Henry's two brothers; Charles John and Arthur James (I); and two sons Arthur James (II) and Dwight. Tom Hood is the son of Arthur James (II).

Numerous donors, including E.P. Charlton, who was the stepson of Arthur James (II), made the library possible. The donors' names are on a plaque in the library. The library has four areas dedicated to honor individuals who made important contributions to the tradition of healthcare in Nevada. This includes the Lounge named in the honor of Dr. Donald Mousel which houses his impressive eyeglass collection. Dr. Mousel traveled to South American to deliver care to low-income natives without access to eye care.

The Reading Room is named to honor Dr. Sandra and Dean Robert Daugherty, who made the History of Medicine Library possible. The Conference Room is named to honor Dr. Owen Bolstad who founded *Greasewood Tablettes* with Dr. Anton Sohn, and the Antique Medical Instrument Display is named to honor Dr. Fred Anderson, who collected many of displayed artifacts. In addition to the 1,000 square feet library, the library also has two offices for faculty. The library is open to the public.

Vol. IX, No. 2, Summer 2000

DR. THOMAS K. HOOD

Thomas Knight Hood was the third child of Dr. and Mrs. A.J. Hood (I). Tom, born in Elko May 13, 1921, graduated from Elko High School in 1939 and entered Pomona College in Claremont, California. The advent of World War II accelerated his education and after three years at Pomona, Tom entered Washington University School of Medicine in St. Louis, Missouri. He enrolled in the Navy V-12 program with an accelerated year-round schooling and earned his MD degree in June 1945.

During his senior year at Washington University he married Irene Segelhorst, a nurse. He served a general internship at the Navy Hospital in Shoemaker, California. He served two years as a medical officer in the U.S. Navy and entered a three-year surgical residency program at St. Joseph's Hospital in San Francisco. After completion of his residency program he returned to Elko and joined the Elko Clinic. Tom served a preceptorship under Dr. George Collett and was certified by the American Board of Surgery.

Dr. Tom Hood's surgical practice was dominated by trauma, with cases generated by highway accidents, railroad accidents and mishaps sent to him from the surrounding ranches. His practice at the Elko Clinic was in association with a number of fine surgeons, including Dr. Hugh Collett, Dr. Matern, and Dr. [Frederick] Owens. This arrangement allowed time for continuing post-graduate education. Dr. Tom was a member of the ama, the American College of Surgeons, the Southwest Surgical Congress, and the Pan Pacific Surgical Association. He served as president of nsma in 1973-'74.

Dr. and Mrs. Hood had three3 children, Victoria, Thomas, and Jacqueline. Thomas died at the age of thirty-six from a melanoma. Victoria is married to a psychiatrist and Jackie is married to a neonatologist. Unfortunately, there is no other descendant in Nevada to carry on the Hood medical tradition.

Tom is proud of his small town background and has been active in community affairs. He is a Rotarian, a Shriner, a member of the Navy League, a member of St. Paul's Episcopal Church, and a director of the Northeastern Nevada Museum. Dr. Hood has also been involved with the development of the Elko Auditorium and Convention Center. He retired from the practice of medicine in 1986 but continued to be active in civic affairs. Dr. Thomas Knight Hood was honored as a distinguished Nevadan by UN and was honored with a Praeceptor Carissimus award by UNSOM, which recognizes outstanding mentoring of medical students.

Dr. Hood's 2002 obituary in the Reno paper states, "Tom will be remembered for his altruism." The editor of the *Greasewood Tablettes* has never known Tom to say "no" when asked to help and was truly dedicated to helping others. In 1993 when the editor was researching 19th-century military medicine at Nevada's seven frontier forts, Dr. Hood volunteered to arrange visits to Forts Ruby and Halleck. He accompanied us on the excursion and helped locate the hospital ruins.

Vol. XIV, No. 1, Spring 2003
Vol. VII, No. 3, Fall 1996

DR. ARTHUR JAMES 'AJ' HOOD (I)

Tom Hood MD

Arthur James Hood (I) was born November 10, 1871. Like his older brothers, he attended Adrian College and in 1903 graduated from the University of Michigan School of Medicine. With his MD degree in hand, he traveled to Elko, Nevada, by train. Arriving in the summer of 1903, he joined his older brother Charles in the practice of medicine. By this means he could repay the $3,000 owed to his brother for his medical education. Their office was a small building facing the Southern Pacific corridor between 4th and 5th Streets. When Charles retired and moved from Elko, Arthur continued to practice, and later associated with a number of partners including Doctors C.W. West, Meritt J. Rand,

Robert P. Roantree, and Charles E. Secor.

About 1928, a new First National Bank Building was constructed on the corner of Fifth and Railroad Streets. Doctors Hood, Roantree and Secor moved their offices to the second floor of this structure. While practicing there they were associated with a number of younger physicians, including Doctors Les A. Moren, Dale Hadfield, and Paul Del Guidice. After the arrival of Dr. George Collett, the Elko Clinic was formed and moved into a building at 946 Idaho Street. Dr. 'AJ' Hood remained a partner in this group until his retirement.

On January 12, 1910, Dr. Hood married Irene Hunter, the daughter of a local cattleman, and took up residence at 431 Pine Street. The marriage produced 4 children, Edith, Charles, Thomas and Patricia. Edith died at the age of 6 from pneumonia. Charles graduated from Stanford University and lived in Elko until his death. Thomas and Patricia followed in order. Patricia graduated and served a residency in internal medicine at Stanford. Her entire medical career was spent in the Bay area and hence is not included in this history.

The first medical problem 'AJ' encountered after arriving in the Great Basin was typhoid fever, which also claimed him as a victim. This disease remained endemic until the water supply for Elko was changed from the Humboldt River to deep wells, along with the Kittridge Canyon Springs. For the first thirty years of his professional life, considerable time was devoted to caring for the somewhat isolated population scattered from the Bruneau River to Eureka. This required travel by horse and buggy, train and automobile.

In 1906, Drs. A.J. and C.J. Hood invested in one of the first X-ray machines in Nevada. As befell many doctors in the early days using fluoroscopy excessively, he received irradiation burns to the fingers of his left hand. The development of skin cancer on his ring finger led to subsequent amputation.

Dr. Arthur Hood felt his most rewarding endeavor was his involvement in securing an adequate hospital for Elko County. In February 1919 his trip to Carson City to lobby to build a new hospital.

One of his greatest disappointments occurred in later life, when he did not hear a telephone ring in the middle of the night. The patient, who was seen by another doctor, turned out to be the former President of the United States, Herbert Hoover. Hoover was one of AJ's idols. During Dr. Hood's last year of life he became debilitated from repeated episodes of hematuria. He died September 18, 1958 from a renal neoplasm.

Vol. VI, No. 4, Winter 1995-96

DR. ARTHUR JAMES 'BART' HOOD (II)

Tom Hood MD

Arthur James Hood (II) was much better known by his friends, family, and associates as 'Bart.' He was the son of Dr. and Mrs. W.H. Hood of Battle Mountain, Nevada, born April 1, 1895. In 1904, his family moved to Reno, where he attended public schools. At the UN he was a member of the Sigma Alpha fraternity, graduating from the University in 1917. He was awarded an MD degree from Stanford University in 1921.

Dr. Hood began a medical practice in Reno, Nevada, in 1921. Although he had no formal internship or residency training, he did post graduate work in Vienna, Austria. Much of his professional activity was in the field of surgery during his thirty-six years of practice. He was on the medical staffs of SMH and WMC, where he served as chief of staff in 1943. Bart served as a consultant for the Nevada Industrial Commission, a position that exposed him to a life-threatening experience when a disgruntled claimant brandished a gun at him. He held a commission as a captain in the U.S. Army and an honorary commission as colonel in the Nevada National Guard.

Bart was a part-time inventor. He devised an innovative barbecue that was powered by an electric fan. With a very small amount of fuel the BBQ could roast a turkey.

Some of these barbecue outfits were manufactured and sold. Bart was a rather large and heavy man physically. He was an inveterate cigar smoker and he loved to travel. He got along well with his many friends. He belonged to the Bohemian Club in San Francisco and was a member of the Prospector's Club in Reno. He was also an Elk, a Shriner, and a member of the Sons of the American Revolution.

His first marriage was rather short-lived, producing no children. His second wife was Elizabeth Charleton whose family was one of the founders of the Woolworth stores. They had two children, Eunice and Arthur James (III). He also gained two stepchildren, Earl Charleton III and Thelma. After the death of Elizabeth (his second wife), Bart married Juliette Toy, the widow of a San Francisco hotel man.

After the surgical removal of a malignant renal tumor, Bart's health slowly deteriorated, and he died in Reno October 23, 1980.

EDITORS' NOTE:

Dr. Bart Hood was Senator Key Pittman's doctor and took care of him during the historical controversy when Pittman died during the November 1940 senatorial race. Dr. Vinton Muller also was present at Pittman's death. Dr. Bart Hood's medical bag is part of the Doctors Hood History of Medicine Library at UNRSOM.

Vol. VII, No. 1, Spring 1996

DR. CHARLES JOHN HOOD

Tom Hood MD

Charles John Hood was born February 23, 1860, in Adrian, Michigan. He attended public schools and graduated from Adrian College. After spending a year or two in Buffalo, New York, studying at the Business College of Bryant and Sons, he returned to Michigan and entered the Michigan School of Medicine, graduating in 1887.

Although he was the oldest in his family, his brother William Henry, one year younger, graduated one year before him in 1886.

Traveling west he set up practice in Spokane, Washington. There he enjoyed a successful period until 1894, when he moved with his new wife Louise to Elko, Nevada. His decision to move may have been influenced by the fact that his younger brother had been practicing in Battle Mountain, Nevada. In 1895, he acquired the medical practice of Dr. Joe Henderson, and in 1903, his younger brother, Dr. A.J. Hood (I), joined him in his practice. They shared an office on Railroad Street in Elko. In 1908, he retired from full time work and moved with his wife back to his boyhood home in Adrian, Michigan. He would occasionally return to Nevada to relieve his younger brother 'AJ' so that he could take further postgraduate training.

As has always been the case, in the 1890s, there were many patients who were unable to pay for medical services. In an attempt to rectify this problem, Charles joined together with two other physicians, Doctors [Samuel] McDowell and [George] Gardner and persuaded the County Commissioners to authorize payment of $125 each month to compensate them for the care of indigents and jail inmates. Prior to that time they had been paid nothing for indigent care. This agreement was continued until sometime in the 1940s.

Much of the care Dr. Hood provided was railroad work. Railroad employees required medical care, and accidents were frequent. The contract physician was assured payment, so the position as railroad surgeon was a coveted one. In 1894, Dr. Charles Hood was appointed Surgeon for the Southern Pacific Railroad. This position was handed down to his brother, and later to the physicians of the Elko Clinic. Typical of the accidents encountered occurred in 1918 when a passenger train carrying a number of Hollanders bound for Java wrecked in the Carlin Canyon. Dr. Charles was standing in for his brother A.J. at the time, and a light engine was dispatched from Carlin to pick him up and transport him to the accident.

In their later years Charles and his wife spent the winter months in Los Angeles. On February 27, 1931, while out for a stroll, Dr. Charles John Hood suddenly became ill. He sat down on a curb and died, presumably from a coronary artery occlusion.

Vol. VI, No. 3, Autumn 1995

DR. DWIGHT 'DUTCH' HOOD

Tom Hood MD

Dwight Lincoln Hood was the second son of Dr. and Mrs. W.H. Hood. He was born in Battle Mountain, Nevada, in 1902. His family moved to Reno in 1904 where he attended public schools. He graduated from the University of Nevada in 1925, earning a BA degree. Dwight attended the medical school at Washington University in St. Louis, where he was a member of the Phi Rho Sigma fraternity. He received his MD degree in 1929 and returned to Reno where he began a general medical practice, holding Nevada State License #1277.

Known by his friends as 'Dutch,' he developed an interest in cardiology, and for many years interpreted ekgs at Saint Mary's Hospital. He was granted a commission as captain in the Nevada National Guard in 1936, and was inducted into the U.S. Army in WWII. Dr. Hood was promoted to rank of colonel during his military career. Active in medical affairs he was a member of the wcms and president of the nsma. He presided over the fifty-first annual meeting of that organization in 1954.

Active in community affairs, Hood was a member of the American Legion, the Prospectors Club, Elks Lodge, Sons of the American Revolution and the Retired Officer's Association.

In spite of a successful professional life, Dwight's family life was tragic. His first marriage was to Florence, who gave him a healthy son named Henry, nicknamed Hanky. One evening Dutch returned from delivering a baby to find that Florence had been killed in a fall down the basement stairs. After this tragic accident Dutch devoted much of his time to Hanky's welfare, but sadly he was killed by an accidental gunshot while duck hunting with his father near Fallon, Nevada.

A second marriage ended in divorce after only a few months. His third marriage to Beulah Brown was a happy one and lasted for years until she died of emphysema near the time of Dwight's retirement. His last marriage was to Keitha. It was a happy marriage, but it was cut short by Dutch's death from emphysema and coronary heart disease October 15, 1979. Keitha survived, living in Reno until her death in 1996.

Vol. VII, No. 2, Summer 1996

DR. WILLIAM HENRY HOOD

Tom Hood MD

William Henry Hood was born on a farm near Adrian, Michigan January 6, 1862, the son of Andrew Jackson and Mary Knight Hood. Although he was the second born son, he was the first to obtain an MD degree and the first of the Hoods to practice medicine in the State of Nevada. After graduating from church affiliated Adrian College he earned an MD degree from the University of Michigan and moved to Battle Mountain, Nevada, to begin the practice of medicine. While establishing himself he worked for a period at a local ranch until securing his professional status. He married Eunice H. Standerwick of Vallejo, California, and fathered 2 sons, Bart and Dwight. The family also included Harry Standerwick, an older son of Mrs. Hood's by a previous marriage.

In 1899, while still practicing in Battle Mountain, William H. Hood was issued license #1 from the Nevada State Board of Medical Examiners. When one of his sons was asked about this, he answered that his father was one of the few doctors in the state who could afford the required $2 fee. He was active in the Nevada State Medical Association and in 1929, was elected president of the Pacific Railway Surgeons—a prestigious professional organization. His wife, Eunice Standerwick Hood, was the first woman to serve on the University of Nevada Board of Regents.

Although he had a rewarding professional career, he became involved in a number of business ventures prior to the great depression. These investments included ranching, a bank, an insurance company, and the Lovelock Mercantile Company. During the depression these businesses lost money and became bankrupt. In an attempt to improve his position, he turned to family members for help and became quite bitter when aid was not forthcoming. There were periods when he refused to communicate with his sons and his brother. In his advanced age, he became chronically ill. He died November 29, 1942.

Dr. William H. Hood developed a reputation as a caring and compassionate physician, and was a well-respected member of the medical community. He well deserved the title of Nevada's Number One Physician.

Vol. VI, No. 2, Summer 1995

EDITORS' NOTE:

A copy of Dr. William H. Hood's BME license #1 issued in 1899 and other memorability of the Doctors Hood are displayed in the Doctors Anton Sohn History of Medicine Museum.

CHAPTER X:
FRONTIER MILITARY MEDICINE

The U.S. Army's presence in Nevada is often overlooked and forgotten. There were seven forts in Nevada in the 19th century and most citizens would be hard pressed to name one other than Fort Churchill (1860-1869), which was built to facilitate soldiers from California heading east to join the Union Army. Later, Camp Nye (1862-1865) was established near Carson City at the mouth of King Canyon to take care of the overflow from Churchill. Fort Henry Halleck (1867-1886) near Lamoille Canyon was built to calm the citizens who were concerned about an Indian threat. Nearby Fort Ruby (1862-1869) guarded the pony express route and was considered the worst military assignment in the West. Today near the town of Paradise Valley, buildings of Fort Winfield Scott (1866-1871) still exist on private property. Fort McDermit (1865-1889) on the Oregon border guarded the Winnemucca-Boise stage route. Fort McGarry (1866-1868) near Summit Lake in northwestern Nevada guarded High Rock Canyon and the Lassen-Applegate Cutoff.

The U.S. Army required military doctors to graduate from an allopathic medical school. As a result, a homeopathic physician had a difficult time enlisting as a physician in the Union Army during the Civil War. Also of interest is that doctors were paid more to serve on the western front. They were paid $125 a month versus $100 in an eastern location. At the same time, a mining laborer received $25 a month. In addition, serving in the West had the benefit of an income from civilian practice. In many locations civilian physicians were not available, and the army felt obligated to serve the public and Native Americans. Most of the military doctors in Nevada were contract physicians with the title of Acting Assistant Surgeon.

Since they had no rank, they had none of the retirement benefits that career officer physicians received. Records from the U.S. Surgeon's Office in Washington, DC, indicate that over seventy military doctors served in the seven Nevada forts during their twenty-nine years of existence. This compares with over 700 civilian doctors in Nevada from 1851 to 1900.

The frontier military doctor had more duties than treating wounded and sick soldiers. At roll call each morning sick call was announced, and doctors were well aware that soldiers took advantage of this opportunity to get out of an assignment. The surgeon also was required to provide a diet to prevent scurvy, which was due to inadequate Vitamin C. As a result, a physician's responsibility was to supervise the planting of a garden at the base and see that the soldiers had a good diet of green vegetables and potatoes, foods that were high in vitamin C.

Hospital or medical facilities were built at all Nevada Forts as the first order of business when construction started on fort buildings. The doctor's responsibility was to oversee the construction of the medical facility. In the following essays, you will read about the presence of military doctors in our state.

BLOOD CURE FOR TUBERCULOSIS
Dr. George Martin Kober

Anton P. Sohn MD

On the 19th-century frontier life was precarious. A common cause of death was infectious disease. Cholera, typhoid fever, tuberculosis, smallpox, diphtheria, and scarlet fever were a more serious threat to Nevada citizens than cancer or heart disease. Infant and maternal mortality rates were high. In addition to health concerns, citizens and travelers in the Great Basin worried about Indian raids. As a result of this threat, forts were established for protection. The presence of the military not only reduced Indian menace, but it brought doctors to the area.

The military doctor not only treated soldiers, supervised the hospital and sanitary conditions, but he also treated private citizens and Indians as well.

In November 1874, George Martin Kober, a U.S. Army doctor treated patients, did anthropological studies on Indian skeletons, built a hospital, studied pathological specimens with a microscope, and wrote scientific articles while stationed at Fort McDermit on the Nevada/Idaho border. Following his stint in the army he became a professor of hygiene at Georgetown University and in 1901, dean of its medical school.

At McDermit in the mid-1870s, he tried an unusual treatment for tuberculosis. Acting Lieutenant Kober, with an interest in hygiene and infectious diseases, read an article about the treatment of tuberculosis advocating daily ingestion of fresh blood from a freshly slaughtered animal. Soon after Kober read the article an emaciated new recruit named Hammond arrived at the fort. A thermometer, recently added to the doctor's armamentarium, revealed fever, while a slight cough and lassitude established for Kober the diagnosis of tuberculosis. Knowing that a steer was killed every other day to feed the troops at the fort, Dr. Kober prescribed a daily pint of fresh blood for young Hammond. The record is not clear as to how long or how frequently the soldier drank the blood, but it does indicate that he regained his health in two months. Probably because he was tired of drinking blood. Much later the bacterial cause for tuberculosis was established and still later an antibiotic was developed, but Kober used fresh blood to effect what he thought was a successful cure.

Vol. IV, No. 2, Summer 1993

MILITARY SURGEON
DR. CHARLES KIRKPATRICK

Anton P. Sohn MD

Charles Alexander Kirkpatrick was nearly twenty-six-years-old and had just begun his own practice of medicine in Grafton, Illinois, when he decided to join a party from nearby Jersey County heading for California Gold fields. He arrived at Mason's Landing at 8:00 am on Monday, April 9, 1849, where he waited until 4:00 pm for a boat to ferry him across the Mississippi River to St. Louis. The long wait gave him opportunity to ponder his decision. He wrote in his diary. "… I will leave it to those who have left home with the intention or without the hope of returning, to describe the feelings with which I left my home and bid a final adieu to the friends that I loved."

When the boat docked he spent the night aboard and in the morning was ready for a day in St. Louis. He found a photographer in the city where he had 'a likeness' of himself taken, and in the evening, visited the theater where he found 'a fair specimen of the immorality of the stage.' He was, "More fully confirmed that virtue did not visit there."

After another day in St. Louis in which he found, "Nothing worthy of note without too much commenting," he boarded the steamer *Timour* in late afternoon for St. Joseph. He took deck passage to begin a 'rough way of living,' but he enjoyed the week of travel on the Mississippi River so much that he wished he had farther to go. Ashore, he found himself in a town of 2,000 inhabitants and a crowd of emigrants, which included men of every description of character, from the honest, enterprising citizen to the lowest, meanest blackguard. He summed up the latter, "Thieves, murderers, liars, Indians, devils, & etc. & etc."

He had another week of waiting until his California-bound companions and the teams from Jerseyville arrived on Friday, April 28. It gave him time to call on the four ladies he had met on the boat, and they greeted him, "As an old acquaintance, and seemed almost as much interested in my welfare as if I had been a relative."

He spent two hours with them and bade them, "An affectionate final farewell and returned to camp feeling that I had enjoyed perhaps my last hours of pleasure in female society," adding, "But so let it be!"

Kirkpatrick was perhaps the most literary member of his company. He was born July 23, 1823, in a log cabin in Pike County. Missouri. An Irish schoolmaster gave him his first lessons in a log house. When he was ten his father, a veteran of the War of 1812, moved to Illinois when the offer of military tract lands to veterans offered a good farm.

After a few years, young Charles became converted to Christianity and followed a missionary, Dr. David Nelson, for one year. In 1841, he enrolled in the first class of the Knox Manual Labor College, working his way through school until he earned a teaching certificate. In 1844, he began a three-year study of medicine with a Dr. Vance in the town of Vermont in Fulton County. In 1847, he attended medical lectures at the Ohio Medical College, and in 1848 commenced the practice of medicine in Grafton, where the Illinois River joins the Mississippi River, not far from St. Louis, Missouri.

It was the first week in May before the Jerseyville Company assembled at Saint Joseph and started on the road. The rains began to fall almost immediately, producing mud through which the men had to struggle. As they came to the 'unbound plain," their emigrant train of seven wagons was joined by another ten teams. Dr. A.R. Knapp of Jerseyville was elected head of the Jerseyville Company.

As he settled into the daily routines of travel, Kirkpatrick wrote of the contrast of goodness and wickedness of mankind and of his own quest for gold. His diary echoes his concerns about the unfairness of deaths he witnessed in accidents and illness. He wrote of his own ills and of the torture of riding in a wagon for ten days when he was too sick to walk. He did not write of medicating himself or of doctoring others. Instead, he wrote of music and dances.

Monday July 23, 1849, Kirkpatrick's twenty-sixth birthday, and a day later some boys from Pike County, traveling in a nearby company, arrived in the Jerseyville camp with a violin and tambourine to provide a hoedown until 11 PM.

We may assume that this was a birthday celebration for the Pike County native and an exception for a weeknight party, because the rigors of trail travel called for early hours, both bedtime and rising. Five days later after a good day's rest on the Sabbath, the Monday morning start on the trail was accompanied by singing. The songs are not mentioned in the diary, but the Pike Company is given credit for producing the first versions of the famous *Sweet Betsey from Pike* and *Joe Bowers*.

On the Humboldt River, while getting ready to cross the desert, the Pike County Boys again visited on August 22, "We had a violin so with this music we had quite a concert." For the next fortnight driving was hard across the sandy desert and up the rocky canyon of the Truckee River, which they were forced to cross numerous times. On September 3, they were at the 'Cannibal Camp' of the Donner Party, where Kirkpatrick took a souvenir tooth from a skull he found. "The view from the summit was worth all the trouble it cost to gain it." He wrote that the roads were unmercifully steep and rocky, and there had been no feed for the cattle, but the travelers admired the huge trees and scenery as they pushed along on their arduous journey.

On September 8, the wagons did not get underway until noon, and that night Doctor Kirkpatrick watched some 'Negro dancing' provided by five men being taken to California by a Missourian, who was also taking 'a lot of little fellows, 'meaning Afro-American lads.

Within a week, Kirkpatrick got his first view of California gold miners work Some of the men in the party couldn't wait and grabbed wash basins to try their luck, with poor results. After a stop at Johnson's Ranch the company pushed on toward Sacramento. Kirkpatrick and 4 other Jerseyville men became sick, and did not reach Sacramento until October 5. For the next two months he was too ill to keep his diary.

On January 1, 1850, he left to rejoin his partners. By this time he had a sign on his tent pole announcing that he was a practicing physician.

He recorded that he sought 'the usual physician's fee for his services which ranged from one half ounce of gold.' In 1850, he was counted in the U.S. Census in Sacramento County.

He moved to Mariposa in March 1850 spending the next winter there, practicing with 'Dr. Bigelow of Boston and others.' In 1859, Dr. Kirkpatrick was in Benicia where he became the U.S. Postmaster. Benicia was a U.S. Army post, an important river port, and for a time the capital of California.

In June 1860, Hutching's *California Magazine* published an article by C.A. Kirkpatrick entitled, "Salmon Fishing on the Sacramento River." It was an account of the decline of the salmon fishery as a result of placer mining. The article is still quoted in environmental studies.

When, he Pony Express delivered the call to California in 1861 for volunteers to fight the Civil War, enlistments began immediately. The first troops were dispatched to the Southwest to fend off an anticipated Confederate invasion. The Third Regiment was recruited in the Gold Country, organized at Stockton and assigned to guard the Overland Route through Utah. The regiment commander Colonel Connor listed Dr. Kirkpatrick as assistant surgeon. The regiment marched from Stockton with a train of fifty-five wagons and three ambulances. Accompanying them were the carriages of officers' wives and their dependents. The column reached Fort Churchill in the Nevada Territory on August 1. Enroute there had been thirty desertions and other such problems reported. While at Ft. Churchill the troops made repairs and reprovisioned. Col. Connor wanted to delay garrisoning Fort Ruby until spring, because "Ruby Valley is a bleak, inhospitable place," but he was ordered to resume the march.

When Connor's column arrived in Ruby Valley on September 1, snow had begun to fall in the mountains. The soldiers were ordered to extra duty, building cantonments under the direction of the quartermaster. The men gathered stone and timber from the nearby mountains for the first buildings at this former campsite, which had served cavalry patrols for the stage and Pony Express.

He rode in the Overland Stage to reconnoiter a site closer to Salt Lake City than Camp Floyd. In October Connor moved his main body of troops to a new site, which was to become Fort Douglas. Meanwhile Assistant Surgeon Kirkpatrick remained in Fort Ruby with 3 officers and 161 men. Kirkpatrick's wife, Mary, remained with him at Ruby. The Kirkpatricks had four children, and while at Fort Ruby, a daughter died in infancy.

In March 1866, Kirkpatrick was mustered out of the army as a lieutenant colonel and moved to Redwood City, California, which had been his wife's home before her marriage. From time to time Dr. Kirkpatrick's medical practice received newspaper attention. In November 1868 a falling tree injured George Rice. Dr. Kirkpatrick treated his fractured skull and amputated his broken arm. Rice recovered to become County Clerk and to find a successful title company. After another accident Kirkpatrick set the broken leg of a carpenter, James Crowe. Crowe later became an undertaker. To keep up with modern developments in medicine, Kirkpatrick returned to medical school and graduated from Dr. Hugh Huger Toland's Medical School in San Francisco.

When Gussie Finger accidently shot Willie McGarvey in the leg with a shotgun, Dr. Kirkpatrick treated him successfully. Later when Gussie was hunting alone he fatally shot himself while crossing a fence. The doctor treated Ned Connors when his arm was broken, but could not save George Rice's thirteen-month-old son when he choked on a screw.

Dr. Kirkpatrick was active in community affairs in Redwood City. He headed a committee to collect money for the victims of the Chicago Fire. He installed the first sidewalk in Redwood City in front of his home. His wife, Mary, was the president of the county's first suffrage society.

Dr. Charles Kirkpatrick became ill early in the 1890s and later suffered a stroke. He died at Saint Luke's Hospital in San Francisco on April 27, 1892. A former patient, James Crowe, handled the funeral.

EDITORS' NOTE:

Reference: Nita R. Spangler, who lives in Redwood City, California. Ms. Spangler has done extensive research concerning the life of Dr. Kirkpatrick, who was a resident of that community for many years. Unfortunately, no photograph of Dr. Kirkpatrick is known to exist.

Vol. IV, No. 4, Winter 1993

WILLOW CREEK MURDER
DR. WILLIAM KENDALL

J.P. Maiden, Winnemucca Historian

In August 1886, word was brought into Winnemucca by stage coach that Andy Kinnegar had been shot and killed in his ranch and store about two miles up from Willow Creek station. Kinnegar was known as a quiet man who lived by himself in the canyon.

Justice W.H. Minor, acting in the capacity of coroner, held an inquest concerning this death. Mr. J.F. Burgan, who had arrived at the Kinnegar place about one-half hour before sundown on August 12, discovered the body. Burgan, together with a man named Miller, found the front door locked, and entered the place by way of an unlocked kitchen door.

Upon entering the house the two men noted a strong odor and found the bloated remains of Andrew Kinnegar seated in a chair. Since the man was obviously long dead, the men departed and went out to report the crime.

Mrs. H.H. McColley, wife of the owner of the Willow Creek Station and ranch testified that on the morning of August 11, an Indian woman named Susie appeared at the kitchen door with a pistol and told her that her husband, One-Armed Jim, had killed Kinnegar. Mrs. McColley, under the impression that Susie had brought the gun in so that Jim would not kill Kinnegar.

Dr. William P. Kendall, the surgeon at Fort McDermit, examined the body of the deceased.

He testified that there was "the track of a ball, either rifle or pistol, extending from the right nasal fauces inwardly, downward and to the left, to a point over the seventh cervical vertebra, producing injury sufficient to cause death."

Immediately Sheriff Fellows began the search for One-Armed Jim. Jim had lost his left hand when a gun exploded while he was shooting. The other Indians stated that he had become resentful, quarrelsome, and dangerous after his accident. He was captured while hiding in the willows along the Quinn River, about five miles south of Fort McDermit. After his capture he was found to have several items that were identified as having come from the Kinnegar place.

The murder trial began on November 19, 1886. Jim pleaded not guilty to the charge of murder. His defense was that a white man had promised him money, if he killed Kinnegar, but was not able to name the man who promised him the money. After fifteen hours deliberation the jury found Jim guilty and sentenced him to be hanged, but prior to the date of execution, 10 of the jurors petitioned the Board of Pardons to commute the sentence. After several petitions and appeals, Jim's sentence was finally commuted to life in prison. Twenty-nine years later, on February 15, 1915, One-Armed Jim died in prison. He was thought to be 109 years of age.

EDITORS' NOTE:

Reference: Historian J.P. Maiden, Winnemucca, Nevada. The original story appeared In Maiden's weekly column in the *Humboldt Sun*. He has kindly given us permission to reprint parts of the article.

"William Pratt Kendal was born September 10, 1858, in Pittsfield, Massachusetts. He graduated from Columbia Medical College in New York City in 1882. Kendall was commissioned as a First Lieutenant in the United States Army in 1885 and served four years at Fort McDermit. He became the last military doctor to serve in Nevada during the frontier days when he closed the hospital at Fort McDermit with the following entry in his daily log: "June 15, 1889—No patients, births or deaths since June 1.

Vol. V, No. 1, Spring 1994

FORT SCOTT IN PARADISE VALLEY
DR. ZETUS SPALDING

Researched by Stephanie Ernaga

Researching history can be exciting because now and then a bit of information appears that will shed light upon a subject that had been at a dead end. Such is the case of Dr. Zetus Newell Spalding, who was only a name until one of his relatives, Gene Sofie of Washougal, Washington, saw Spalding's name in my book on frontier military medicine and contacted me by email. Until then, there was no face or information to go with the name Dr. Zetus N. Spalding was listed in the records of Fort Scott, which is near Paradise Valley, as acting assistant surgeon during 1865. His personal military records were missing from the National Archives in Washington D.C. (Only in recent years has increased government security prevented pilferage of historical records from the National Archives.)

The following is the story of Dr. Zetus Newell Spalding as related by Mr. Sofie. The earliest known ancestor of Zetus Spalding was Edward Spalding, who came to America in 1619 with Sir George Vardley. Descendants of Edward lived in Vermont, where Zetus was born on August 13, 1819, in Albany, Orleans County, Vermont.

When Zetus was seven-years-old the family moved to Ohio, finally settling in North Norwick on the Sandusky and Mansfield Railroad. After elementary education, at the age of twenty-one, Zetus commenced the study of medicine at the Norwalk Academy under the preceptorship of Dr. Hugh F. Prouty in Monroeville, Ohio. He completed his medical degree six years later at the Cleveland Medical College in 1846, Dr. M.C. Sanders moved to Roxana, Michigan. Zetus was restless, and like thousands of Americans, he headed west to pursue his golden dream.

He arrived in Sierra County in California on August 12, 1852, and worked in the mines for three years before going into the mercantile business in St. Louis, Sierra County. In July 1857 he lost everything that he owned in a disastrous fire. He married seventeen-year-old Mary Ann Brown from Sussex, England, in August after the fire.

With a new wife to support he found a way out of his financial predicament by volunteering for the U.S. Army. The Indian Wars in the West were heating up, as was the Civil War, and the U.S. Army was searching for doctors at an attractive salary of $100 per month.

After his military service Dr. Spalding returned to Susanville, California, where he became county physician, coroner, and public administrator for Lassen County. He established a pharmacy called Spaldings Drugs in Susanville with another relative, A.C. Neal. The Pharmacy was still in existence until recent years. Dr. Spalding had eight surviving children, losing several to diphtheria. At least two great granddaughters still live in Susanville. His brother, Noah, lived at Eagle Lake in Sierra County from 1873 until 1880.

Dr. Spalding died on May 17, 1898, apparently drowning while fishing in the Susan River. He is buried in the old cemetery in Susanville. Much is still unknown about Dr. Spalding's life and career in Susanville, but slowly the pieces of the puzzle are coming together.

Vol. XII, No, 2, Fall 2001

NEVADA'S FRONTIER FORT HOSPITALS

Owen C. Bolstad MD

FORT HALLECK'S HOSPITAL

The monument marking the location of Fort Halleck is on the fence line between the Chivelar Ranch and the '71' Ranch owned by Pete Marble. The Chivelar Ranch is on the right near the Halleck Fort site.

The best-preserved part of the fort is in an old cottonwood grove, with lengths of stone foundations up to thirty inches wide and forty feet long. According to maps of the old fort, these ruins represented outbuildings. A search for remnants of barracks and officers' quarters led us to a pasture west of the trees, and after some time we were able to find foundations of a number of buildings. There had been two hospitals built at Halleck, the first being condemned as having inadequate rooms, kitchen, and treatment facilities. We located both the old and the new hospitals across the fence to the east side on '71' Ranch. We located the foundation of the old hospital and used a metal detector to find some flat metal and a broken pitchfork. We found some fragments of medicine bottles and other artifacts. The new hospital is about 500 feet on a hill to the north. Two of the maps in the National Archives in Washington DC, show the new hospital in the wrong location. There were new factory-made bricks and a recent fire on the site, but there were old stone foundation blocks suggesting an earlier structure. The medical artifacts, broken bottles, and vials were a help to locate the hospital foundation. There were also horses where the ruins were located.

FORT SCOTT'S HOSPITAL

On November 2, 1993, at the Fort Scott site, we scattered peacocks when we entered the gate, and were met by Freda, a small deer with a bell, and Susan Kern and son Davey. The fort's buildings are by far the best preserved of any we have visited. The Kerns are living in one of the original officers' quarters, and the barracks were being used as a barn. Across the parade ground are the remains of a building.

This building was largely intact until a few years ago when half of the roof collapsed. We had a map of the old fort and were able to locate the site of the hospital. Then, Susan exclaimed, "I never noticed that before," and pointed out a straight line of obscure rocks about 30 inches wide and forty feet long. They had been driving across those rocks for years, which were the foundation front wall of the old hospital.

Fort McDermit's Hospital

Referring to a map of the old fort, we located the site of the hospital, some five hundred feet up the hill from the tribal headquarters. A bulldozer had recently leveled this site, and all that remained were two stone and concrete pillars.

Fort Churchill's Hospital

Fort Churchill's Hospital has been well cared for after an initial period of neglect, and the wpa had done renovation and preservation. The block stones that were the fort's hospital walls are well known and well preserved in the Nevada State Park.

Vol. V, No. 1, Spring 1994

CHAPTER XI:
UNUSUAL, BUT THIS IS NEVADA

SERIOUS CASE OF OVER STUDY
DR. T. PARRY TYSON

Richard Pugh, Former NSMA CEO

The following is the story of an incident that occurred in 1923 in Wadsworth, Nevada, involving the shooting death of Dr. Thomas Parry Tyson. (Various sources indicate his name was J. Perry Tyson; we are using Nevada Board of Medical Examiners' records that indicate his name was Thomas Parry.) My thanks to Dr. Tyson's grandson, Jerry Tyson of the San Francisco Bay Area for permission to share his thoughts on this event and to Pierre Hathaway, Jerry's Carson City relative who provided interesting details and valuable newspaper clippings of this incident.

Dr. T. Parry Tyson, a well-known and respected Reno physician, seemingly became a raging 'madman' and 'maniac' when he went on a shooting rampage while 'holed up' in the Wadsworth Bazzini Hotel in 1923. Tyson was born in 1866 and received his medical training at the University of Pennsylvania School of Medicine. He was licensed in Nevada in 1905 and became chief autopsy surgeon for Washoe County,

In a front-page headline dated February 1923 the *Reno Evening Gazette* reported the tragedy in which Washoe County Undersheriff J. W. Carter killed the doctor with a .45 caliber automatic pistol.

It was reported that Dr. Tyson had traveled to Wadsworth from San Jose for the expressed purpose of encouraging Paiute Indians in the area to rise up against white settlers. While it is not entirely clear why he wanted to do this, Jerry Tyson speculates that he apparently was distraught because the fishing grounds were being deprived of water.

This was due to the 1915 Newlands Reclamation Project and construction of the Lahontan Reservoir and Derby Dam. Dr. Tyson's grandson also suggests the doctor may have become disturbed at the numerous Indians he suspected had been murdered by white settlers. "Dr. Tyson may have had good reason to be sympathetic to the Indian cause," said the grandson in a recent letter to Mr. Hathaway.

The *Reno Evening Gazette* headlines, "On Battle With Posse–Former Nevada Physician Dies in Pistol Duel–Maniac Endangers Lives of Citizens–Arrest Sought When Attempt Made to Get Piutes (sic) to Wipe Out Whites–J. Perry Tyson Holds Force of Officers at Bay in Wadsworth Hotel."

There were numerous attempts by Washoe County Sheriff J.D. Hillhouse, Deputy Sam

Kearns, Deputy J. W. Carter, Justice of the Peace W.D. Ingalls, and the owner of the Bazzini Hotel to persuade the doctor to surrender, but nothing worked. Kearns and Carter were thought to have used tear gas but were not successful in getting the doctor to give up. They injected chloroform through the keyhole into Tyson's room, a tactic suggested by Physician Samuel Lees Joslin who was on the scene. The tear gas and chloroform worked to get the disturbed physician to vacate the room, but it led to his being shot and killed by Carter. Evidently Carter spied Tyson through a knothole taking dead aim at Kearns and shot first, possibly saving Kearn's life.

Dr. Tyson had moved from Reno to the San Jose area in 1917, but he returned to northern Nevada yearly. On one of his visits in 1922, he was arrested on a 'lunacy charge' and was paroled into the custody of his son, Howard Tyson, who took him back to the Bay Area.

The doctor returned to northern Nevada on February 12, 1923, and stayed at the home of a longtime friend, Mrs. Zeigler, who saw him off to Wadsworth two days later. She later commented to investigators that he appeared normal at the time.

The *Gazette* commented that Dr. Tyson had been studying psychiatry and was planning on writing a book on the subject and that he became 'unbalanced as a result of studying psychiatry which pertains to healing mental diseases and to which he was devoting his energies in writing.' The *Reno Evening Gazette* headlines on February 18, 1923, state, "Tyson's condition was a result of over study."

The *Nevada State Journal* reported that Dr. Tyson's body was sent to the Ross-Burke Mortuary in Reno on February 17 to await instructions from the family in San Jose. "Tyson became mentally deranged and endeavored to have the Indians at Wadsworth annihilate white settlers," commented the writer of the article. "He had been of unsound mind for a long period...although at times he appeared lucid."

Howard Tyson interred his father in a 'beautiful columbarium in Oakland.' It is possible that all the facts of his father's death may never be known. There was a brief investigation, but no evidence was ever presented to disprove anything other than Dr. Tyson being shot in the line of duty by Under Sheriff Carter.

Jerry Tyson states the family will continue to think of our ancestor as an eccentric but good person who was sincerely trying to help our native brothers.

EDITORS' NOTE:

A few days after we published the article on Dr. Tyson, we received a call from longtime Reno Surgeon Ed Cantlon. Ed remembers vividly the day Tyson was killed in February 1923 in the Nevada House. Ed was twelve at the time and living in Wadsworth on the family ranch. He was sent down to get the mail from the Columbus Hotel, which is across the railroad tracks from the Nevada House. Authorities would not let anyone cross the tracks because a 'crazy man' in the Nevada House, wanted to kill white folks for what they did to the Indians. Joe Bazzini owned the Nevada House, also called the Bazzini Hotel. Ed was in the post office when Tyson was shot. He didn't hear the gunshots. According to Dr. Cantlon, the hotel was eventually sold to Joe Bianchini who became a longtime patient.

Vol. XIII, No. 2, Autumn 2002

RESURRECTED LUCKY BILL
DR. BENJAMIN KING

Gary Ridenour MD

Bill Thorrington lived in the Carson Valley in the 1800s. He was a giant of a man and his friendly nature, and generosities were as well-known as his skill at gambling and drinking. He made fast money playing three-card Monte and Thimblerig. Sometimes these winnings included land and personal property, which always led to bad feelings. Two of these losers were John and Enoch Reese, founders of Mormon Station in Genoa. Their debt was an astonishing $23,000 and they were forced to turn over "their ranch, all hay and grain from that year, eight yoke of oxen, ten head of horses, sixty head of hogs, seventy chickens, the blacksmithing tools, the dry goods and groceries in the store, all furniture and cooking utensils, the claim to the Eagle Valley Ranch and Old Emigrant Road."

Bill accepted the payment and promptly moved to the ranch with his girlfriend Mary Lamb, a woman from the Sacramento saloons, while his wife and son tried to ignore the situation and live in Genoa near Honey Lake on Barter Creek. Henri Gordier began to build a herd with some of the finest cattle in the valley. One day in 1858, a neighbor, Sol Penin, noticed a rider passing by his ranch and recognized him as Lucky Bill Thorrington, a gambler he used to know in the early Placerville days. Bill, in his usual pleasant demeanor, asked where Gordier could be found for he was interested in buying some cattle from him. Sol gave him directions to the Gordier place and Bill rode away. Two days later he stopped by Perrin's place and told him that he would be sending some men back for the cattle that he had purchased.

A month or so later neighbors of Gordier heard that the Frenchman had suddenly sold out and left for parts unknown.

A man named Asa Snow was living on the old Gordier ranch. Soon John Mullen and William Combs joined Snow and began working the ranch. This was not the first time that someone had given up life in the West and gone home, but Gordier's freeloading alcoholic brother began writing to the neighbors inquiring about Henri's welfare. Mullen and Combs quietly disappeared into the Nevada night. In late April, a group of vigilantes from Honey Lake were out looking for some Pit Indians, who were said to be rustling cattle. The campfire talk turned to the missing Frenchman, and one of the men suddenly remembered that he had heard a single gunshot about the time of Gordier's disappearance. He was sure that it was the one that did in the Frenchman.

A search party turned up ashes, partially burned clothing and blood near Willow Creek, and later, they found Gordier's body in a deep spot in the river, weighted down with a rock. A hastily formed jury in Honey Lake found both Mullen and Combs guilty of murder in absentia. Snow and Lucky Bill were found guilty as accomplices. Snow was soon apprehended. He was uncooperative, and while the posse was questioning him he was "accidentally" hung, dying of "unknown heart problems." Lucky Bill and Combs were caught and tried in the Sides and Abernathy barn near Genoa. Unfortunately, Bill's appointed lawyer was named Reese, and was probably related to Enoch and John Reese. During the trial a gallows was built and both were found guilty and sentenced to death.

The impending hanging interested a Dr. King, who was experimenting with galvanic cells. He told the curious that he was interested in reviving the dead by electrical shock, feeling that if electricity could take a life, it might be able to restore it. Dr. King talked to Bill, and he agreed to the plan, providing that he was properly buried after the experiment.

Bill was hung near the Clear Creek Ranch from the back of a wagon. He sang "The Last Rose of Summer" and was a gentleman until the end. Combs confessed that he and Mullen had killed Gordier, and that he knew nothing of Bill Thorrington.

William Combs was hanged for the crime near Janesville. Dr. King quickly retrieved Bill's body and successfully revived him with electrical shock. Ten years later witnesses from Colorado reported that Bill Thorrington was living in that state. The vigilantes opened Bill's supposed grave and found only rocks. Lucky Bill Thorrington never returned to Nevada and supposedly died of old age. Dr. King left town soon after the episode, and we hear no more of him or his electrical devices.

EDITORS' NOTE:

References: George and Bliss Hinkle, "Sierra-Nevada Lakes," Reno: University of Nevada Press, 1987; Michael J. Makley, 'The Hanging of Lucky Bill," Eastern Sierra Press, 1993; Norm Nielson, 'Tales of Nevada," Tales of Nevada Publication, 1991; and Phillip I. Earl, "Lucky Bill got lucky again...or did he? *Nevada Appeal*, 1982. Vol. VII, No. 3, Fall 1996

TROUBLED DOCTOR
DR. FREDERICK HUGO WICHMANN

Eileen Barker, UNSOM Pathology Department Manager

Perhaps one of the most colorful physicians ever to have practiced in Nevada was Dr. Frederick Hugo Wichmann. Born in St. Louis, Missouri, about 1874, he worked his way through the University of Illinois, graduating in 1902. After obtaining his degree, he enlisted to serve with the insurgents in Cuba, and helped them fight their battle for independence. When American forces invaded Cuba during the Spanish-American War he befriended General Frederick Funston. After that war, General Funston became the commandant of The Presidio in San Francisco and served there during the great earthquake and fire of 1906.

Dr. Wichmann followed the rush of gold prospectors to the far north during the Alaska Gold Rush. He practiced medicine in the arctic region but returned to California when an patient shot him because he was enforcing sanitary regulations. practiced medicine in Lovelock, Nevada, in 1905, moving later to Reno where he soon got into trouble.

On September 10, 1906, he was accused of performing an illegal operation on a patient named Lily Benson. The poor woman died of 'blood poisoning' on October 14, 1906.

While awaiting trial on the abortion and murder charges, he was accused of assaulting another women named Ethel Fine, and as a result of that accusation, the woman's brother, Fred Fine, shot Dr. Wichmann in the arm. The wound became infected, and the doctor's life hung in the balance for some time when 'septic poisoning invaded his entire system.' His attending physician advised amputating the infected arm, but eventually the physicians decided to remove two inches from his ulna, while authorities awaited the outcome of Dr. Wichmann's life threatening infection.

On December 5, 1906, the State of Nevada indicted Wichmann for the murder of Lily Benson. By March 1907 following a trial during which the stepmother of Lily Benson testified as to Lily's 'wild ways,' Dr. Wichmann was acquitted of the charge. Within a year Dr. Wichmann was almost continuously in trouble with the law. There was another abortion charge. He threatened his tailor with a gun. He was involved in street fights and named in assault charges. In May 1910, following a charge of disturbing the peace and carrying an unlicensed firearm, Dr. Wichmann signed a deposition admitting to excessive gambling and drinking, and promised to keep peace in the future.

On October 6, 1910, Dr. Wichmann was arrested on a charge of murder, following the death of yet another patient, Mrs. Emma Ross, after an alleged abortion. The first-degree murder trial, which began on February 1, 1911, was sensational. District Attorney William Woodburn and Assistant District Attorney M.B. Moore prosecuted the trial with Judge French presiding. The defendant's attorneys were Judge W.W. Jones and young attorney Patrick A. McCarran, who would later become a powerful United States Senator. Numerous well-known citizens of Reno were called to testify at the trial.

Dr. Sidney King Morrison, the county physician was called to give expert testimony, as were Drs. George McKenzie, Albert Heppner, Mulchyor Wise, Charles Edward Mooser and A. Parker Lewis. Dr. A.W. Wullschleger and Dr. O.J. Johnstone were called to testify, as was Mr. William Cann of Cann's Pharmacy, who testified regarding a prescription for ergot and quinine. Nurse J.A. Talbot, of the Talbot Sanitarium was called, as was the Reno Chief of Police Burke. Mr. J.P. O'Brien of the Groesbeck and O'Brien

Undertaking Firm testified. Mrs. Rosalie Saunders, manager of the Nortonia Apartments on Ridge Street where Mrs. Ross had resided after her arrival from Los Angeles, was called to the witness stand.

Dr. Oscar Johnstone, from the bacteriology department at the University of Nevada, to whom Dr. King gave the body organs removed from Mrs. Ross for his examination gave his opinion. Mrs. M.A. Lissak of Saint George's Hospital also related her experiences.

Dr. Wichmann was not without support in the community, for he was considered handsome and quite affable, as well as having considerable medical ability. Many of his friends testified in his behalf. The trial came to a sudden conclusion when the Assistant District Attorney, in his closing argument, asked for a conviction of involuntary manslaughter, rather than the original charge of murder. After adjournment, the jury went to dinner at the Riverside Hotel, returning to the Jury Room at 7:30 pm. It took just two hours and forty-seven minutes before the foreman of the jury, Mr. E.H. Roctor, read the verdict of guilty. Sentenced to eight years in prison, Dr. Wichmann served just eighteen months of his term when five hundred petitioners were able to get the parole board to release him in September 1912. His medical license was revoked on May 1, 1911, and Dr. Wichmann left the state.

On April 14, 1916, The *Reno Evening Gazette* reported that Dr. Wichmann had gone to Mexico to serve in the army of Francisco (Poncho) Villa. It was further reported that he had created a sensation when he appeared half dressed in the streets of El Paso, Texas, with the story that he had been sentenced to be shot at sunrise by Villa, but had made his escape.

Nothing further is known concerning the fate of this colorful character from early Nevada, a man who seemed to attract trouble wherever he went.

Vol. IV, No. 2, Summer 1993

LYNCHING AND RELYNCHING
DR. EDWARD S. GRIGSBY

Dr. Edward Shepard Grigsby graduated from Hahnemann Medical College, a homeopathic school in 1894. Like many doctors he was attracted by mining excitement and the need to supplement his income from medicine. He went to Nome, Alaska, and later to various locations in Nevada (Bullfrog, Rhyolite, and Tonopah). He was licensed in Nevada in 1905. He formed a partnership with Dr. Patrick J. McDonnell, a graduate of Johns Hopkins Medical School, who arrived in Tonopah in 1910.

While practicing in Rhyolite, Dr. Grigsby was called to attend Jim Arnold's lynching by the citizens of the mining camp. Arnold was tried by the mob for killing Jim Arnold Joe Simpson in Skidoo. The doctor's car got stuck in the sand and he didn't get to Skidoo in time to save Arnold, but he was associated with one of the most famous lynching stories of the West. Simpson's dead body was 'strung up' several times, as everyone in the town wanted a picture of the lynching and the citizens obliged by a reenactment of the incident, including for the sheriff when he arrived. The story is a favorite 'western,' and no doubt the doctor told it as many times as other spectators of the 'reenactment' did.

Vol. XVII, No. 2, Summer 2006

PARKING ON THE RAILROAD TRACKS
DR. A.P. LAGOON

Dr. A.P. Lagoon came to Ely in about 1900. As a result of a Spanish-American War accident, he had a peg leg, but he hunted, fished, and could drink anyone under the table. He claimed that he could do more with his peg leg than most men could do with two normal ones. Dr. Lagoon performed operations on kitchen or library tables.

One night in the saloon, several men were boasting about how much weight they could carry. The doctor claimed that he could carry 500 pounds of sugar across the main street from corner to corner–chuck holes, mud and all. The saloonkeeper took bets and banners were made for the event. Five hundred pounds of sugar were delivered from the big mercantile store at Lane City and the contest was on. Ten other men tried to carry the sugar and failed. Lagoon's turn came and he won and collected the money.

In 1908, he bought a new car for trips to Ruth, Reipetown, and Kimberly. About a month later, coming down from Ruth, he stopped on the railroad tracks while he and his three friends made a comfort stop. An ore train came around the curve and smashed the car. Nevada Northern Railroad refused to pay for the car since it was stopped on the tracks, and no one occupied the car at the time of the impact. Doc claimed that the engineer would have had plenty of time to see them had he not been asleep. Railroad officials met with their lawyers and told Doc that he had no case. Lawyers said he could tell his story in court. Then Nevada Northern Railroad's lawyers asked, "What about the other three men involved? What would they say?" Just then Lagoon piped up and said. "They'll swear to anything I say—they were drunk!"

He so charmed the railroad investigator that they awarded him money for a new car, and he promptly spent his new fortune entertaining them.

EDITOR'S NOTE:

References: *The Nevada Bicentennial Book* by Elgas, Paher et al. A search of the files at the Nevada State Board of Medical Examiners' office shows no evidence of licensure for Dr. Lagoon in the years between 1900 and 1908 *Practiced Medicine in the Territory and State of Nevada from 1855 to 1957.*

Vol. III, No. 2, Fall 1992

FRONTIER JUSTICE AND MALPRACTICE

Kirk V. Cammack MD

When I came to Las Vegas in 1960, just out of my surgical residency, the town was still a frontier gambling town. Five or six years later, with the arrival of Howard Hughes, it began to develop into a cosmopolitan city of over a million people—as it is today. Besides the 'mob element' gamblers in the valley, there was a group from the western states and gambling ships off the coast of California who had migrated to Nevada where what they were doing was legal. It wasn't very long after coming to Nevada that I operated on one of the Texas gamblers who had been shot in the abdomen. The man survived. This Texas gambling contingent had come to Nevada to escape a dangerous war going on in the Dallas area with their competition. This is when I met Golddollar. He stood six feet-six inches, and had all gold teeth. He had been the first black man to be admitted to the Professional Rodeo Cowboys Association. He was the bodyguard of a leading Texas gambler in Las Vegas. He was very quiet, but at the same time a very intimidating man.

One day, Golddollar was in my office waiting to be seen, when this agitated family came in yelling and upset over the death of their daughter.

He had come into the trauma area after having been beaten up and overdosed. It had been difficult to make a diagnosis of her situation, and eventually she died. The family was irate, and threatened to sue me, screaming and hollering, and disrupting my office. 1 took them into my private office to try to talk with them, but to no avail. They left the office, saying that they were going to see an attorney that day and file a lawsuit against me for malpractice.

Golddollar (such nicknames were common in the western states) asked my receptionist, "Who were those people? And what was the problem?" She briefly explained the situation to him. He asked for their address, and she gave it to him (it was hard to deny Golddollar anything.) Several days later, I received a call from the family, saying they wanted to talk to me. 1 told my office staff that I didn't want to hear any more of their vituperation, and to do what they had to do. One of the office staff said, "They are nice now, and they want to talk to you." When I got on the telephone with them, they were very calm and apologetic for their behavior and said, "We are not going to sue, and you should not be concerned with us at all." At the end of the conversation they said, "Thank you very much for your help, and would you please tell Mr. Perry Rose (Golddollar's real name) that we are not going to sue, and there will not be any problem." Their attorney called me to reassure that there would be no lawsuit and to inform Golddollar.

The next time he came into the office, I asked Golddollar what he said to those people to get them to decide not to follow up with a lawsuit. He rolled his eyes sideways and shrugged his shoulders and said, "Doc, I don't know what you're talking about." I never mentioned the subject again. It was a malpractice suit avoided by Frontier Desert Justice, Texas style.

Vol. IX, No. 4, Winter 1998-9

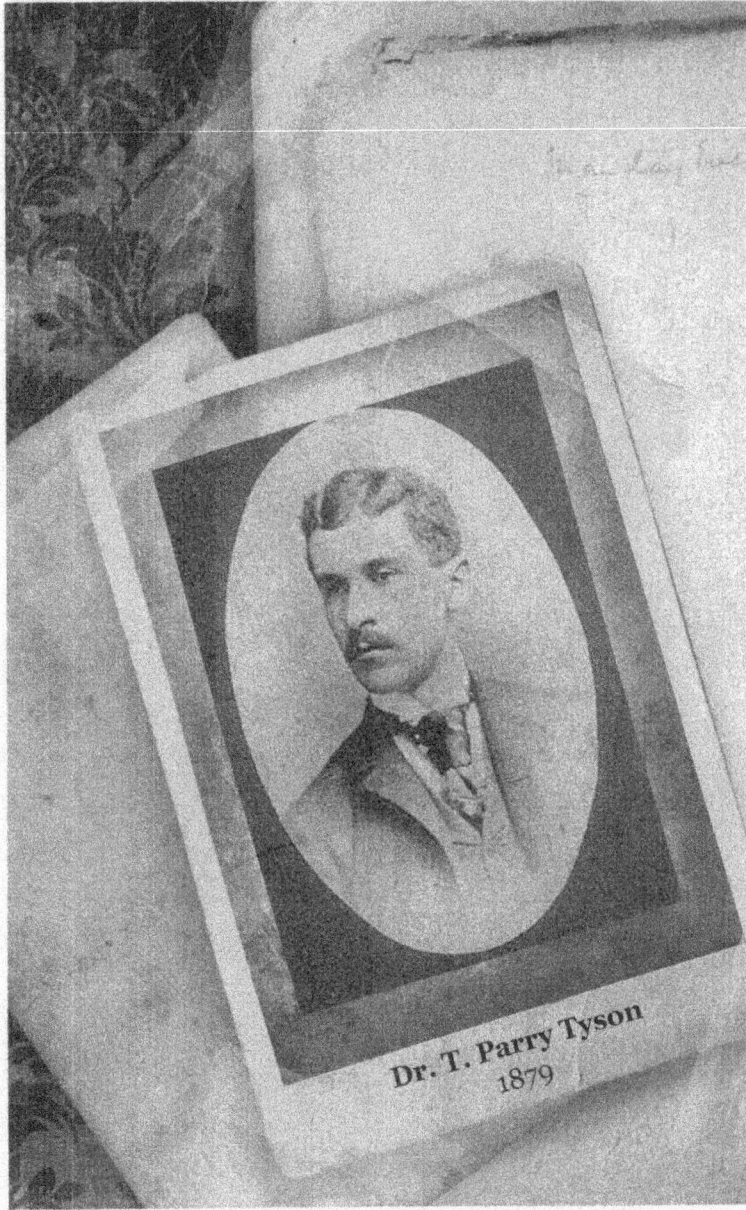

Dr. T. Parry Tyson
1879

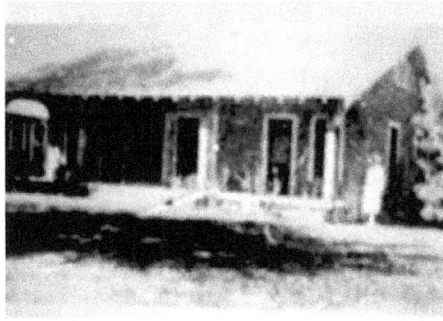

CLARK CO. INDIGENT HOSP. 1931

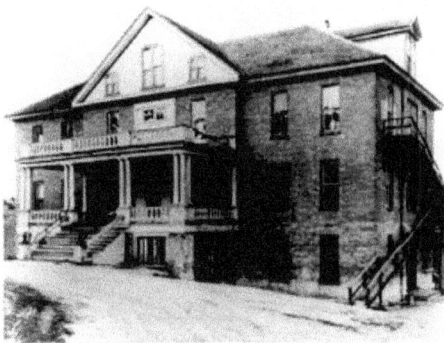

Saint Mary Louise Hosp.
Unk Date

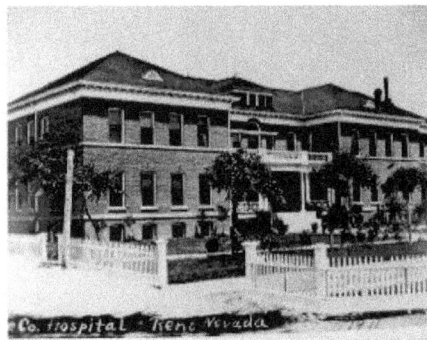

Washoe Co. Indigent Hosp.
1906

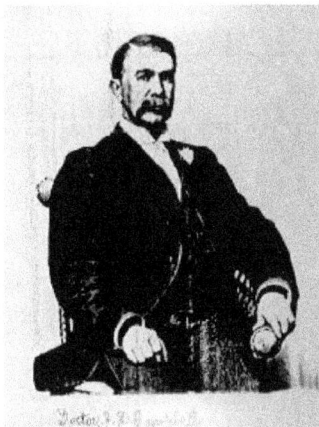

Dr. John Campbell, 1920

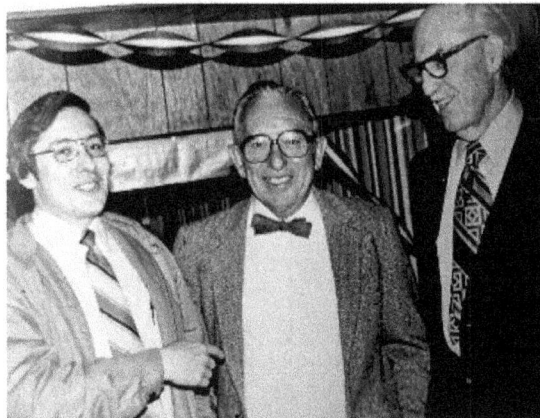

Lt, Drs. M. Dingacci, A. Dingacci
F. Anderson, 1979

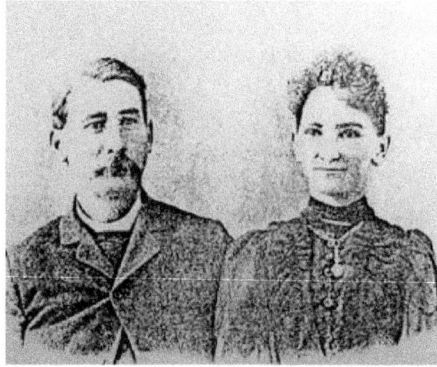
Dr. Weaver & Wife, 1880s

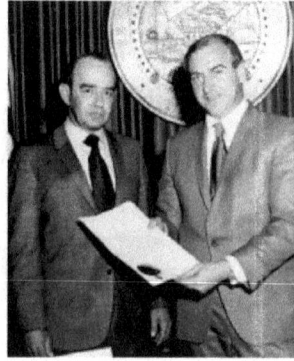
Dr. V. Elliott & Gov.
M. O'Callaghan, 1971

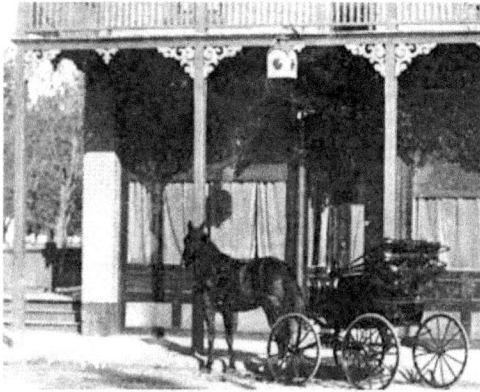
Reno Hosp. 1915

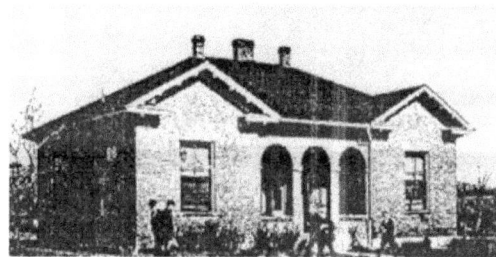
Univ. Nev. Hosp. 1920

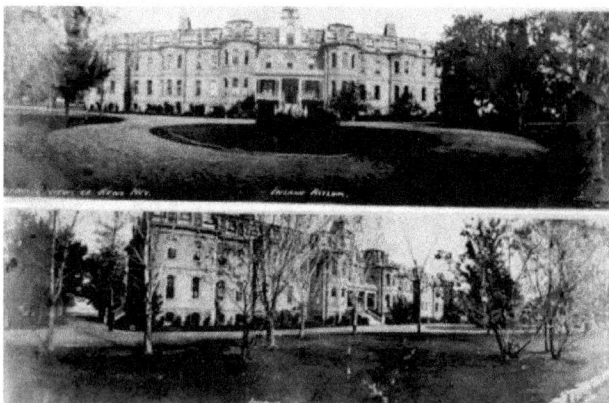
Nev. State Hosp. for the Insane 1882

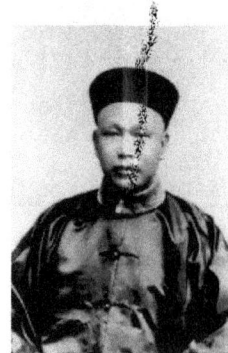
Dr. Wai Tong, 1899

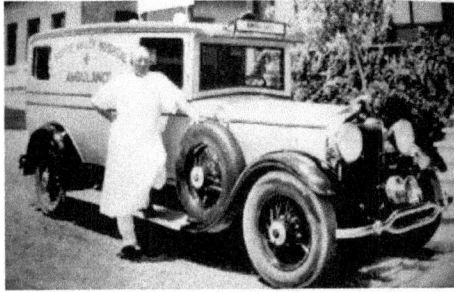

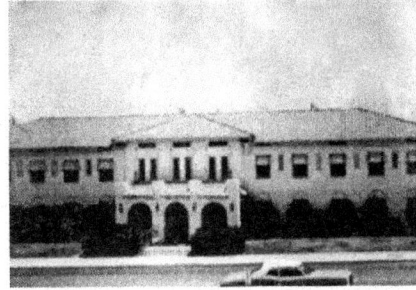

Steptoe Hosp. Ambulance, 1930s   Las Vegas Hosp. 1976

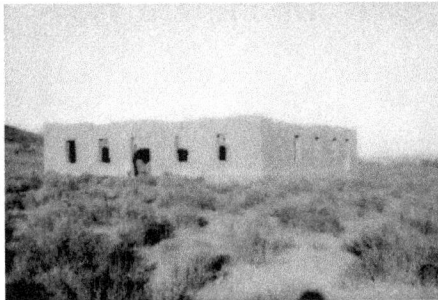

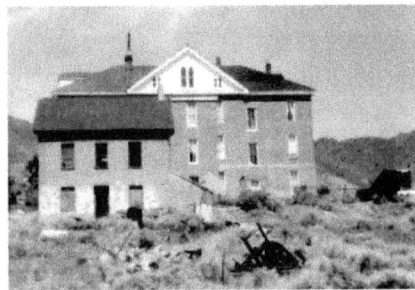

Ft Churchill Hosp. 1994   St Mary Louise Pest House, 1939

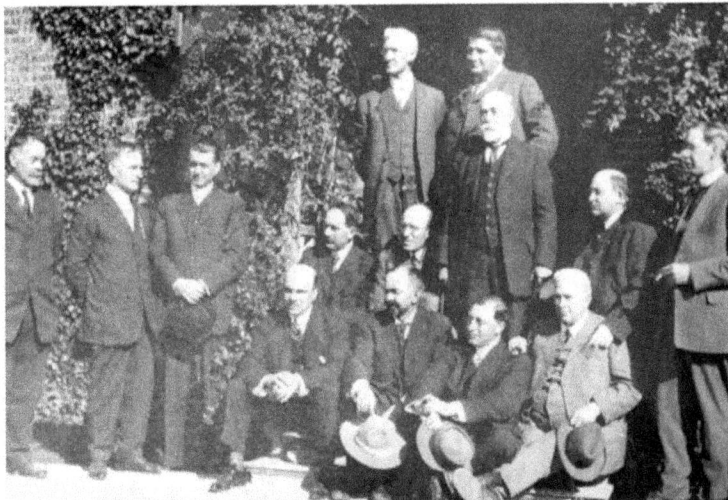

1909 in Front of Saint Mary Hosp. Reno

Standing Left (left to right): E.B. Gregory, Raymond St. Clair, R.L. Robinson
Seated Front (left to right): R.K. Hartzel, W.H. Hood, W.L. Samuels, J.E. Pickard
Standing Back (left to right): John Lewis, George McKenzie
Standing Middle: Henry Bergstein
Seated Middle (left to right): M.R. Walker, S.K. Morrison
Standing Right (left to right): Parker Lewis, M.A. Robinson

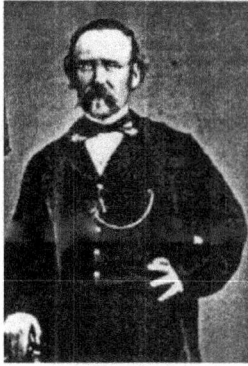

DR. A. TJADER, 1860s   DR. V. MULLER, 1950s   DR. P. STARR, 1950s

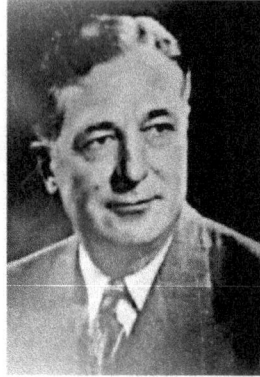

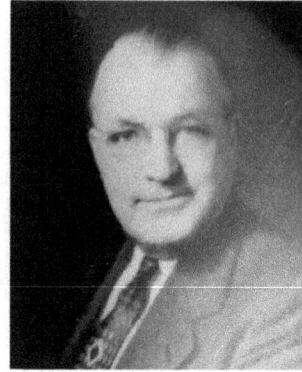

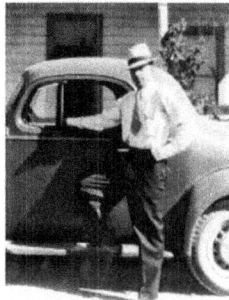

Dr. G. Sylvain
1937

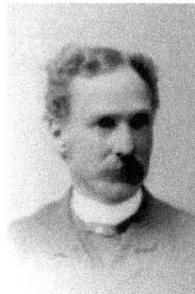

Dr. G. Thoma
1890s

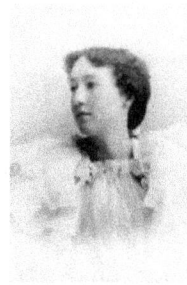

Dr. A. Thompson
1900

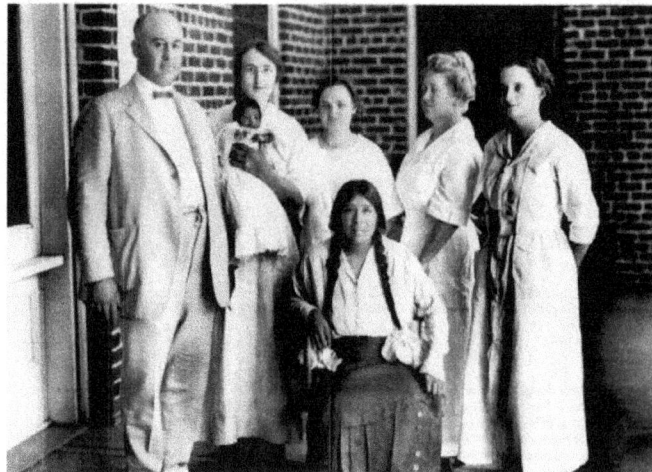

Dr. J. Gerow, Nurses Holding Baby, Indian Mother, 1920s

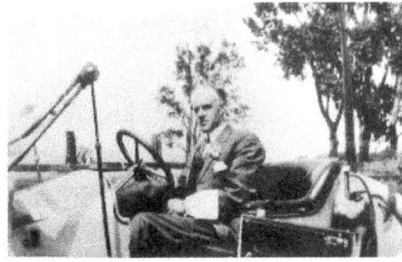

DR. D.M. MACLEAN 1920S

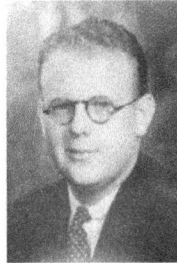

Dr. K. Maclean
1950s

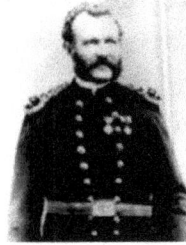

Dr. S. Lee
1901

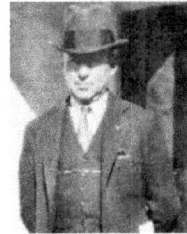

Dr. R. Martin
1930s

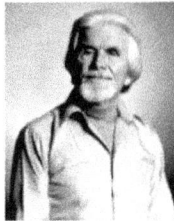

Dr. L. Miller
1979

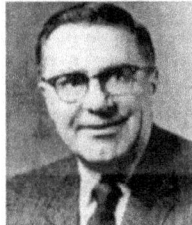

Dr. L. Moren
1954

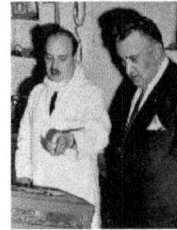

Dr. G. Smith & W. Baring
1960s

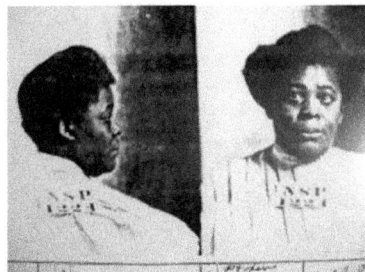

Mollie Harrison, 1908

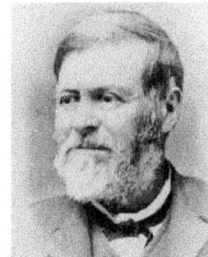

Dr. Z. Spalding, 1980s

ACRONYMS AND ABBREVIATIONS

AB	Nevada Assembly Bill
AED	Alpha Epsilon Delta (pre-med. honorary Fraternity)
AHEC	Area Health Education Center
AIDS	Acquired Immunodeficiency Syndrome (See HIV)
Ama	American Medical Association
Anesth.	Anesthesiologist
BA	Bachelor of Arts
bio.	Biography
BME	Nevada Board of medical Examiners
ca.	Circa or approximately
CCMA	Churchill County Museum and Archives
CCMS	Clark County Medical Society
CME	Continuing Medical Education
COS	Chief of Staff
Derm.	Dermatologist
ENT	Ear, Nose, and Throat (otolaryngologist)
ES & LVN	Eagle Standard and Lahontan Valley News
GW	Greasewood Tablettes
NNHSM	Northeastern Nevada Historical Society and Museum
NNM	Northeastern Nevada Museum
HEW	U.S. Department of Health, Education and Welfare
HIV	Human immunodeficiency virus (The cause of aids)
IM	Internal Medicine
IOOF	Independent Order of Odd Fellows
LV	Las Vegas
NBME	National Board of Medical Examiners
NHS	Nevada Historical Society
NLM	National Library of Medicine
MSU	Michigan State University
NSA	Nevada State Archives
NSJ	Nevada State Journal
Nsma	Nevada State Medical Association
OHS	Oregon Historical Society
OB/GYN	Obstetrics/Gynecology
Ophth.	Ophthalmologist
Ortho.	Orthopedics
Path.	Pathologist
Ped.	Pediatrician
PR	Public Relations
REG	Reno Evening Gazette

RMSF	Rocky Mountain Spotted Fever
SMH	Saint Mary's Hospital, Reno
SMLH	Saint Mary Louise Hospital
SOM	School of Medicine
TB	Tuberculosis
T&A	Tonsillectomy and Adenoidectomy
UCADS	Univ. of Calif. Anthropology Dept. and Smithsonian Inst.
UCLA	Univ. of California, Los Angeles
UCSF	Univ. of California, San Francisco
UKSOM	Univ. of Kansas School of Medicine
UN	Univ. of Nevada
UNLV	Univ. of Nevada, Las Vegas
UNR	Univ. of Nevada, Reno
UNSC	Univ. of Nevada Special Collections
UNSOM	Univ. of Nevada School of Medicine
UNSOMS	Univ. of Nevada School of Medical Sciences
USC	Univ. of Southern California
WCMS	Washoe County Medical Society
WHO	World Health Organization
WICHE	Western Interstate Commission of Higher Education
WMC	Washoe Medical Center (Renown Medical Center)
WPA	Works Progress Administration, (A Relief Agency 1935-'43)

ACKNOWLEDGMENTS

To acknowledge those who have helped us over twenty-five years to chronicle the history of Nevada medicine that spans over one hundred and fifty years is a daunting task. Read the one hundred and two essays written by forty-one essayists in this book and count the number of mentioned people who helped and supported us in our task, and you will understand why the authors do not stand-alone. We might fail to mention a few because the number of helpers would rival the size of the unr phone directory. However, at the top of the list is Dr. Owen Bolstad, who in 1989 helped start the Great Basin History of Medicine Program. He enthusiastically endorsed and co-founded the oral history program, which today has over one hundred and twenty-recorded interviews in the School of Medicine's library. Not only did he supply important material, and he was also there at every junction as a friend.

As to the staff of Greasewood publications, we want to particularly acknowledge the contributions of Eileen Barker, Lynda McClellan, and Teresa Garrison. Eileen was the UNRSOM Pathology Department Manager when the Great Basin History of Medicine program started. Not only did she format and type manuscripts, but more importantly, she provided ideas and became a significant part of the driving force in recording Nevada's history of medicine. She diligently did research, oral histories, and travelled the state. She visited outlying county recorder offices to research the names of doctors who applied for a Nevada license to meet the 1875 registration requirement.

Teresa and Lynda came later in the game to the department of pathology, but their contributions held the program together and provided much needed support and ideas. We cannot over emphasize the importance of their help, and we could not have functioned without them.

Another person whose influence reaches back to the beginning of the history of medicine program is Dr. Kristin Sohn, author and unheralded copy editor of all of our publications. The authors wish that they had her knowledge of the 'King's English.' Also, my wife. Arlene Sohn helped with support and important suggestions.

In addition to above named individuals, several others were with us at the beginning: Phyllis Cudek and Rick Pugh cheerfully undertook interviews and supplied valuable essays for *Greasewood Tablettes* and Greasewood Press publications; Martha Hildreth and Bruce Moran from unr's history department gave needed support and creditability to our program, and Tom King supplied guidance on starting our oral history program.

Just as important was Dr. Rod Sage, whose literary genius was the hand that edited many of our essays and provided research and essays on a number of subjects important to the history of medicine in Nevada.

There are a number of individuals who heard of our efforts to record Nevada's history of medicine and supplied research, photographs, and essays for *Greasewood Tablettes* and this book.

These include: Director Caroline Ford, Susan Ervin, Sandy Klimek, Dr. Kirk V. Cammack, Lori Romero, Dr. Bill Simpson, Anne McMillian, Dr. John M. Davis, Dr. Donald S. Kwalick, Dr. Tom Hood, Cynthia Pinto, David Prosser, Betty Bianchi, Lynne D. Williams, Annie Blachley, Janet K. Holmes, Chelsea Isom, Julie M. Schablitsky, Raymond A. Grimsbo, Professor John P. Marshall, Ryan Davis, Professor Elmer R. Rusco, Dr. Gary Ridenour, Albert R. Paulson, Phillip I. Earl, Lee Mortensen, Linda Dufurrena, Anita Watson, Robert Ellison, Gerald Ackerman, and Toni Mendive.

We thank the sixteen individuals who brought to our attention their family history. These include: Walter McMeans, Carole Flaxman, Beatrice Rey, Mabel Baker, Margaret Duensing, Denise Cervantes, Richard A. Sumin, Jerry Tyson, Gay Metcalf, Charles T., Wegman, Barbara Parish, Allen Roberts, Kimberly Campbell, Linwood W. Campbell, Gary Tinder, Gary Tjader, and Karen Roberts.

We are indebted to Dr. Sanford Barsky and Dr. Marcus Erling UNRSOM pathology chairmen, who allows us to publish *Greasewood Tablettes* in the pathology department. Finally, we were guided by the knowledgeable hand of Guy Rocha, who knows everything there is to know about the history of Nevada, including medicine. We appreciate his counsel, which reaches back to the 1989.

INDEX

www.ingramcontent.com/pod-product-compliance
Lightning Source LLC
Chambersburg PA
CBHW061324190326

41458CB00011B/3884